HER DIFFICULT CHOICE

Decisions. choices. Manipulation.
Survival. Opportunities. Hope.

By

Johnnie Hogg Beatty

Johnnie Hogg Beatty

RED FLAGS
MENTAL ABUSE
TRAUMA BONDING
DESPAIR
HOPE

DEDICATION

For Kimli Ann Beatty Peckham, this book is for you.

and

To all the Ladies that developed Stockholm Syndrome along the way, and to those who had spouses who were predators and survived.

ACKNOWLEDGMENTS

LISA FERNANDEZ And ILLARA FERRIS FOR THEIR HARD WORK TO MAKE THIS BOOK HAPPEN!

TABLE OF CONTENTS

CHAPTER ONE

The morning light crept across the orphanage floor in a thin, trembling ribbon, the kind of light that made dust look like drifting snow. I came into their lives on what must have seemed like another ordinary morning, when Amy crossed the dining hall with a dish towel still in her hand, thinking only of chores and the quiet hum of the day. Her mind was on the familiar rhythm of the morning, the clatter of dishes, and the soft murmur of voices, but something at the door caught her eye: a small, bright shape resting against the threshold.

Amy, one of the caregivers, opened the wooden door, and then, through the screen door, she spotted the yellow color of my clothing. At first, she thought it was the sunlight spilling across the floor. She looked again, and her breath caught in her throat. Then she exclaimed loudly, "Come quick, come see what someone left at our door!"

Chairs were pushed back from the table, and everyone dropped what they were doing to see what the excitement was about. The Headmaster, Becky, peeked around everyone and sighed, then said in a soft whisper, "We are being blessed. Someone left us a beautiful little baby. What does the note say?" she asked.

Amy held a small note fluttering slightly in the breeze. It appeared to have been torn from a notebook.

Her fingers trembled as she began to read, "Please love and care for my sweet Tera. I can no longer care for her. She needs goat's milk twice a day. Other baby foods, she can have whatever you have. She is 3 months old. Signed, Her Mother."

Becky picked me up and wondered where I had come from. Yet, in that moment, it no longer seemed to matter. I became theirs that day to love and care for. No one called the authorities. No one wanted the interference of the cold machinery of the outside world that might take me away. I had become their obligation, their duty, and they felt bound to that commitment.

"It's my turn to hold her! It's my turn to care for her!" whispered Amy, as she reached for me, hoping that Becky would let go of me.

The caregivers began to knit, began to sew, and began to line up for a chance to hold me. Their hands moved with tenderness and purpose, each stitch and each touch carrying the warmth of a love that had already taken root.

Mary Sue leaned in close, her voice barely above a breath. "She is so tiny. Look at those little fingers."

"She has your nose, Becky," Janie teased softly, and a ripple of quiet laughter moved through the room.

"She has nobody's nose but her own," Becky replied, her voice tender but firm. "And from this day on, she has a home."

Later, I began to crawl. I no longer fit in the basket that I had arrived in, but Amy found a crib in the attic that looked just right for me. She cleaned the crib and whitewashed it to make it look new. The ladies all joined together and quilted a blanket for me, each square sewn with care and quiet affection. Amy took the discarded basket out to the wash house and removed all the linings and cloths to clean them. When she lifted the tiny little mattress, she found a torn piece of notebook paper, a little smudged and wrinkled, attached to another paper.

Amy carefully smoothed it out, her hands suddenly unsteady. "Oh, my goodness," she whispered, mostly to herself. "It is Tera's birth certificate." She read it again, just to confirm to herself what she was holding.

"Unity Hospital," she read across the top of the paper. Then she saw my name.

They now knew that my name was Tera Lynn Riff. Reading further down, Amy saw that my mother's name had been marked through with what looked like charcoal. It was completely unrecognizable.

Amy began to shout, "Look what I found! Come quick!" She waved the document in the air, back and forth, trying to get everyone's attention.

Amy held on to the piece of paper, waiting for Becky, pressing it close to her chest. I imagine she must have thought, now we have something of Tera's, something that gave her a name, and the thought settled deeply within her heart.

Becky took the paper carefully, as though it might dissolve in her hands. She read it twice in silence, then looked up.

"Unity Hospital," she said quietly. "Her name is Tera Lynn Riff."

The room went still.

"Riff," Amy repeated slowly, as if the word needed time to settle. "It suits her somehow, doesn't it? Like a little song."

Becky folded the paper with great care and placed it against her heart for a moment before handing it back to Amy. "Keep this safe. It is the only piece of her story we have."

"What do we do with it?" Amy asked.

"We keep it," Becky said simply. "We keep it, and we keep her."

They would deal with everything else themselves. No one needed to know. Nothing else mattered to them. They had somebody they all could love and care for. After all, my mother had brought me to them.

The morning chores were almost finished. Becky had been sitting at the small hand-carved desk nestled in the bay window. She always enjoyed resting in that corner, where she could look out across the yard and let her thoughts wander. From there, she watched the cows swish their tails back and forth, mostly to keep the flies from landing on their backs. Beyond them, the horses raced across the open field as if something important were about to happen. There was a strange energy in the morning air, something she could not quite place. Then a faint cry from the back finally jarred her out of her thoughts. It was Amy with startling news. In an instant, the ordinary day was transformed into a joyful, happy one, with all the ladies joining the children in laughter and sharing juice, their voices filling the orphanage with warmth and excitement.

***

A few months later, I had two little teeth coming in at the bottom. I was running a slight fever, and now the caregivers knew the reason. Amy called out to the dining room, "Someone please bring me a wet cloth to bring the fever down. Tera is too warm." Immediately, caregivers Mary Sue and Janie came to the rescue, hurrying in with concerned faces and gentle hands. It was not long before I was calm and fast asleep, the cool cloth resting against my tiny forehead while the women watched over me with quiet relief.

"Now let's prepare for the holidays," said all. Christmas was here, just three more days away.

Becky spoke up to let the ladies know that funds were very short and only the most necessary gifts could be bought for the children. There were fifteen children, all under the age of ten, and all looking forward to Santa. It was important that the older ones received a gift, not meant to slight us babies, but we would simply have to wait our turn for Santa.

A warm bottle at night would have to do until next year. Even as she spoke, Becky felt the weight of the decision, knowing how much joy even the smallest gift could bring.

Amy and her roommate, Julia, were sent to get gifts for the children who were over one year old. There were ten in all. Amy was given $30.00 to get something for each of the children who were expecting Santa to come. It was not much, but they were determined to make every dollar count and bring smiles to as many little faces as possible.

Becky had the children decorate the Christmas tree that the village had provided. Those little children went to bed very pleased and happy with their decorating skills, their eyes still shining with excitement from the ornaments and ribbons they had so carefully placed. They were unaware of the shortage of money. They were warm and happy anyway, and for Becky, that brought its own kind of comfort.

The next morning, there was a knock at the orphanage door, but when Amy opened it, there was no one there. She looked out into the cold morning air and saw no sign of anyone. Then she spotted a package resting at the door and brought it inside, noticing that it was addressed to me.

Amy, filled with excitement, opened the gift to find a wrapped, soft, fuzzy white pony that could walk by pushing a button. She carefully pulled the little pony out of the box, noticing its beautiful head and long mane, and that it was wearing a lacy red cap with its ears pulled through. Everyone laughed, cheered, and danced around, all excited that I had received a gift. The room seemed to burst into life with their delight, and for a moment, every worry about money and shortages disappeared.

I got a gift after all, even though my birthday was still two months away, and I was in the group that would not be receiving a Santa gift. Someone had remembered me, and that small act of kindness touched every heart in the room.

"Who could have sent it?" Janie asked, turning the box over in her hands, searching for a return address that wasn't there.

"Someone who knew," Amy said quietly.

"Knew what?"

Amy looked down at me, already reaching for the fuzzy white mane with wide, delighted eyes. "That this one needed to be remembered."

No one spoke after that. They simply watched as I patted the pony's soft nose over and over again, laughing a breathless, gummy laugh that filled every corner of the room.

As I grew, my fondness for horses grew with me. A toy horse was better than a doll, better than anything else to me. From the very beginning, it seemed as though something deep inside me had already claimed them as my own.

***

The next year, Santa brought me a pair of bright red cowboy boots, just the right size for my tiny feet. I wore those boots to bed for months, refusing to part with them even at night, until the weather became too warm to continue wearing them. I cried when I was told they had to come off. Instead, the boots were allowed to go to bed with me, so I could cuddle and hold them until morning. I would often fall asleep with one tucked beneath my arm and the other pressed close to my chest, as if they were the most precious treasure I owned.

The orphanage owned a stable with several horses. Some were used to cultivate and plow the fields, since all our vegetables came from our own ability to provide. Some of the horses were trained to give riding lessons to the town children who could afford to take lessons. I would often slip away from my caregiver, and that day it was Amy, peeking around the corner as I watched the stable boys care for the horses. My eyes would widen with wonder as they brushed their coats until they shone and spoke to them in calm, familiar voices. I began to hope and dream that someday I could also go to the stables and brush the backs of the horses, or at least one of the ponies. I also saw the mucking, but I did not desire to be part of that.

One of the older stable boys, a lanky teenager named Will, caught me watching one afternoon.

"You want to brush her?" he asked, nodding toward a chestnut mare named Daisy.

I stepped forward so fast I nearly tripped over my own boots. "Can I?"

Will handed me the brush with a grin. "Slow strokes. She likes to know you're not in a hurry."

I nodded seriously, placed my small hand flat against Daisy's side the way I had seen Will do, and began. The mare exhaled slowly and dropped her head.

"See that?" Will said. "She trusts you already."

That was all I needed to hear.

Finally, at age six, I was allowed to take lessons too. Becky thought that since I was older, I could go to the stables alone. My excitement could hardly be contained, and from that day forward, the stables became my favorite place in the world.

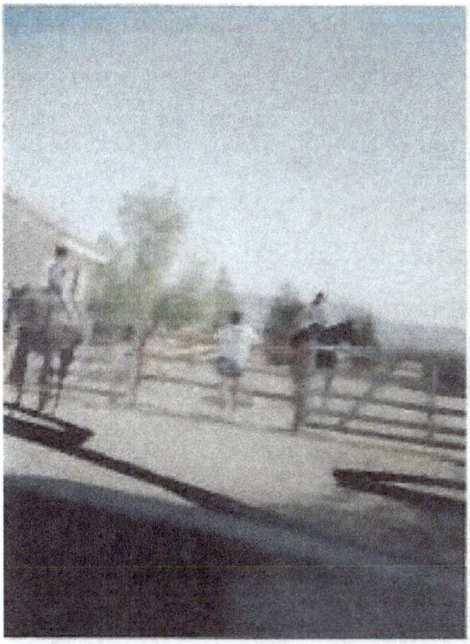
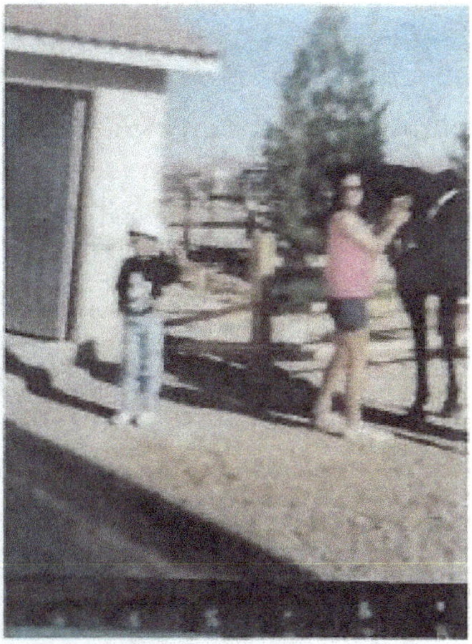
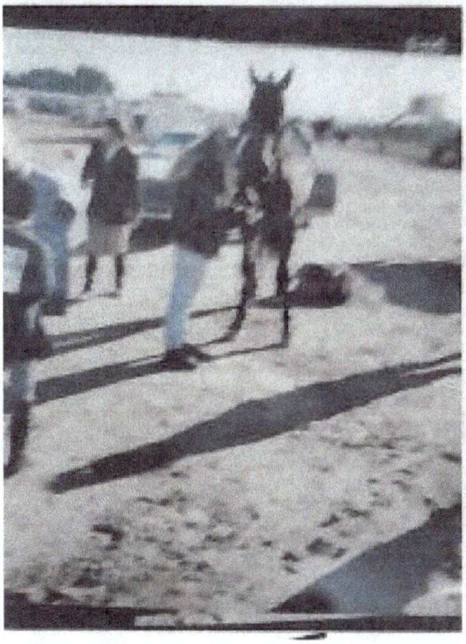
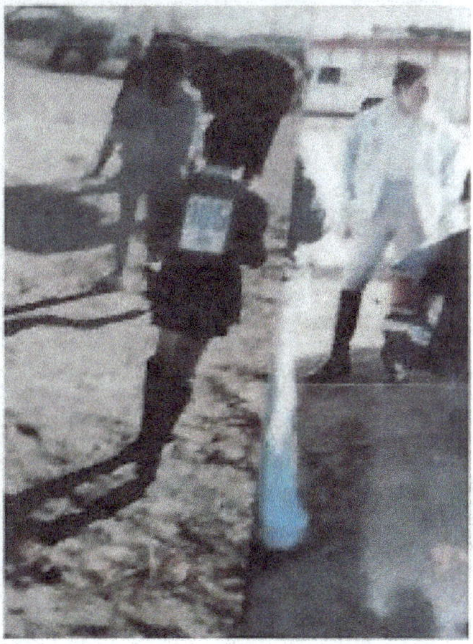

Soon, I was able to help the trainers with the town children who were learning to ride. Therefore, I was included with the trainers, learning all I could about caring for the horses and, ultimately, for the children too. There were days when I would move the horses the wrong way, or at least not in the direction that the trainers were indicating. I tried so hard to do everything right, yet sometimes confusion clouded my efforts.

Then one day, Becky noticed that my eye drifted inward, not quite like a lazy eye, but enough to cause concern. Maybe that was the reason I was not seeing what the trainer was saying when he was signaling to me. A quick visit to the doctor told Becky what she already suspected. I needed a minor operation to correct that muscle. So, at six years old, a minor operation corrected it. However, at the same time, the doctor found that the sight in that eye was not as strong as the sight in the left eye and, therefore, would cause some reading problems. I was given "granny glasses" to wear that looked absolutely adorable on me. I sometimes complained that I felt dizzy, but I continued to wear them faithfully.

Becky would often take me and two of my friends shopping at the consignment shop downtown. It was where everyone would go to find the perfect dress for all occasions. I always picked out the ones that looked very western in style, dresses and outfits that would match my cowboy boots. I always appeared dressed perfectly, no matter the occasion, with a touch of that same little cowgirl spirit that had grown with me over the years. I was now into wearing my second pair of red boots, having outgrown the others.

Leaving the consignment shop, I spotted a flyer posted on the front window. The poster showed a guitar slung over the shoulder of a cowboy wearing a black cowboy hat. The lady standing next to him in the poster was holding a microphone, and the beautiful boots she was wearing caught my attention immediately. Then I read:

ONE NIGHT EVENT ONLY.

COUNTRY STARS TIM McGRAW AND FAITH HILL

TICKETS AVAILABLE INSIDE.

What I did not know was that Becky had gotten four tickets to the event to surprise the girls who had excelled on their language exam. I was one of them. I stood and stared at the poster, dreams floating through my mind, thinking, *I will never get to go see them.*

It was getting late in the evening, and I was beginning to wonder why we were still in town this late. Becky had bought me perfectly fitted red jeans with a matching red shirt. They both matched the red boots I was wearing, and Becky had me try them on. Once I looked into the mirror and saw the wonderful fit, I did not want to take them off. My long brown hair hung to my waist, and with the bright red outfit and boots, I felt transformed. Becky did not insist on my changing back into my shopping clothes. I felt like a princess, all dressed in red and standing in front of the poster, my heart full of wonder and dreams I had barely dared to imagine.

Becky took me and the other two girls by the hand and walked us over to the theatre where the event was advertised. It was for that very night. I wanted so badly to beg to go, but I was far too polite to ask. My heart beat faster with every step we took toward the building, and I could hardly keep my eyes off the bright lights and the large poster at the entrance. Becky walked up to the ticket agent, handed over the four tickets, and said, "These are for you girls to go and enjoy the musical. You have earned it." Then Becky took a red felt cowboy hat out of the bag she was carrying and gently placed the hat on my head, smiling at the look of wonder that instantly filled my face.

I was still puzzled as to what was happening, as this had never occurred before. No one from the orphanage had ever gone to a concert. For a moment, I simply stood there, staring in disbelief, trying to understand that this wonderful surprise was truly meant for me and the others. I was important to Becky! Then the realization swept over me, and I danced around Becky, hugging her and tugging on her arm with excitement.

I was so overwhelmed with joy that I was not sure I could contain myself without screaming and yelling at the top of my voice. I was going to see the stars and hear them sing. To me, it felt as though one of my brightest dreams had suddenly come to life.

The auditorium was huge, with steps leading high up toward the top, what seemed to me like over fifty feet in the air. The vastness of it left me breathless. Quickly, we found seats for the four of us to sit together. We were midway to the top, but we could still see clearly, and to me, it felt like the perfect place to be.

I listened, clinging to every word in every song as if there would never be another chance to hear it again. Each note seemed to settle deep within my heart, every lyric becoming something I wanted to remember forever. It was an unforgettable night, a night I knew I would relive in my dreams again and again.

Becky had not yet noticed that I was no longer in my seat. The girl beside her tugged at her sleeve.

"Becky. Becky, look."

Becky turned, and her breath caught. There I was, halfway down the aisle in my red boots, walking with the quiet certainty of someone who had already made up her mind.

“Lord help us,” Becky whispered, but she was smiling.

Becky had just introduced me to a whole new world. During the singing, I decided that I wanted to see the stars up close. Before anyone could stop me, I was halfway down to the stage, moving with the fearless excitement only a child could have. Tim McGraw looked up and saw this beautiful little girl, all in red, walking toward the stage. He stopped his song and gently asked, “Are you here to see me?”

I looked at him, my eyes wide as they caught the sparkle of the stones on his jacket, and answered honestly, “No, I am here to see her.” I pointed toward Faith Hill.

The auditorium burst into laughter.

Faith Hill was still a newcomer to the music world, not yet widely known to everyone, which made my innocent answer all the more charming.

Everyone in the auditorium laughed so loudly, but Tim McGraw was smiling with joy. There was no offense in his expression, only delight. He reached down, took me by the hand, gave me the microphone, and said, “Join Faith in this next number. I bet you have a beautiful voice.”

When it was over, Tim McGraw crouched down to my level and said, “You’ve got something, little one. Don’t ever let anybody tell you different.”

I looked at him with the calm seriousness only children can manage. “I know,” I said.

The laughter that followed was warm and long, and it followed me all the way back up the aisle to where Becky stood, still shaking her head and dabbing the corner of her eye with her sleeve.

It was an event that I will never forget. The magic of standing so close on the stage, the warmth of the lights, the laughter of the crowd, and the kindness of the singers all settled into my heart as a treasured memory. We all went home that night, filled with excitement and eager to tell the others what had happened, knowing that this story would be told again and again within the walls of the orphanage.

***

Soon, I was of age to go to public school. Since I excelled in languages, I learned to speak Spanish very quickly and, in turn, would help my roommates learn to speak it as well as I could. I was excited to attend school, eager to learn more than what had been taught at the orphanage. A new desire had crept into my thinking and settled firmly in my mind. I wanted to sing!

I joined the church choir, along with two of my other orphanage friends. It was not long before there were music and harmony filling the dining hall at every meal, our voices blending together and bringing a new kind of joy into our daily routines.

Most of us children were taught in the orphanage grounds until we became thirteen. The only contact we girls had with boys was with the field workers, and sometimes with the delivery men who brought store supplies. We would exchange a few words, but nothing more.

The orphanage was twenty-two miles from the nearest town, and therefore, we had little outside contact with others. I was looking forward to seeing boys and girls who might be different from what I was used to. I carried a quiet curiosity about the outside world, wondering what it would feel like to be part of something beyond the familiar walls of the orphanage. I would soon find out.

On September 15th, the first day of public school, I walked out to meet the school bus along with four of my roommates. We were all so excited and felt so grown up to be going to a school outside the orphanage. Our laughter and chatter filled the morning air as we waited, each of us filled with nervous excitement and anticipation.

I got on the bus last, and the only seat still available was beside a red-haired young boy. I was not sure if I should sit or wait until he invited me, so I stood there for a moment, unsure of what to do, my hands clasped together as I hesitated.

Finally, he said, "My name is Chase, and if you would like, you may sit with me."

I smiled timidly and sat down, my heart beating just a little faster as I settled into the seat beside him.

They rode in silence for a moment, the kind that wasn't quite uncomfortable but wasn't easy either.

"Is this your first time on a school bus?" Chase asked, not unkindly.

"Yes," Tera admitted. "Is it that obvious?"

"A little." He glanced at her boots. "Nice boots, though."

I looked down at my red boots, then back at him. "Thank you. I've had them since I was two."

Chase raised an eyebrow. "These same ones?"

"No," I laughed, and it was the first real laugh I had given all morning. "I've grown since then."

Later that day, I was invited to join two other girls playing volleyball. I had never seen the game before and decided to try to join in. There was no television in the orphanage, so everything about it was new to me. At first, I watched carefully, trying to understand the rhythm of the game, then slowly began to follow along. I soon got the hang of it and was really having a great time, laughing and moving with the others, when suddenly a ball came crashing over the net and struck me on the side of the head. I had not been watching the ball because, out of the corner of my eye, I happened to see Chase walking across the campus. My attention had shifted to him without my even realizing it.

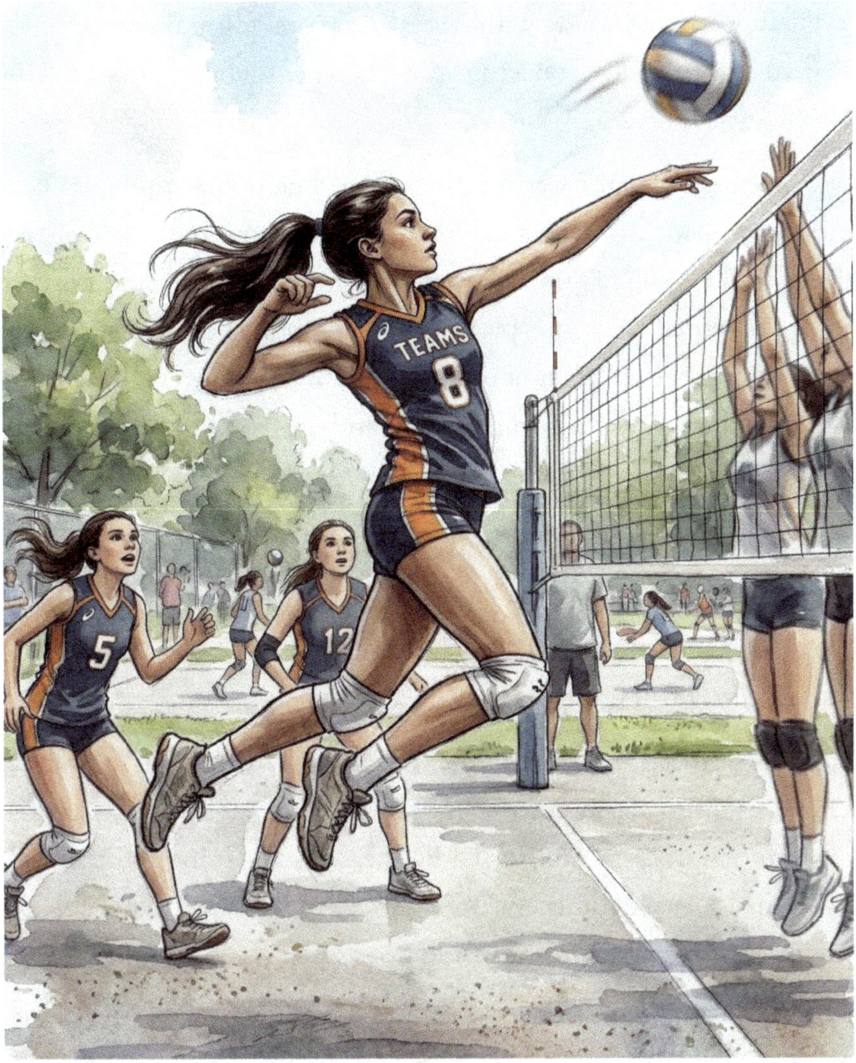

I came to from my fall, lying on the ground with Chase trying to place his coat under my head. The world around me felt distant for a moment, voices blending together as I tried to focus.

"What happened?" I asked softly.

Chase answered, along with several girls speaking at the same time, their voices filled with concern. "You fell. The ball hit your head. The school nurse is coming."

Three hours later, I was on the bus heading home with a swollen knot on the side of my head. I had recovered from the worst of the dizziness, but I still felt unsteady, as though the world around me had not quite settled back into place. Every bump in the road seemed to echo through the tender spot on my head. "When you get home, put a cold compress on the swollen knot and go rest," the nurse had explained gently.

A week went by.

I seemed to be all right. At least, that was what I kept telling myself. It was not until I tried to race my horse, Molly, that I recognized I was not as well as I had thought.

Molly seemed to know that I was not all right, too. She balked at the stall, not wanting to let me put the saddle on her. The usually gentle horse shifted uneasily and tossed her head, as if sensing something I myself had not yet admitted. After several tries, I was finally able to mount Molly to ride, but she would not move.

"What's going on, Molly?" I inquired, confusion and frustration creeping into my voice. By now, the trainer had noticed that I was having trouble getting Molly to let me ride.

"I think you had better go inside and let another day go by before trying to ride," the trainer, Bob, said in a calm, knowing tone. "That is called horse sense."

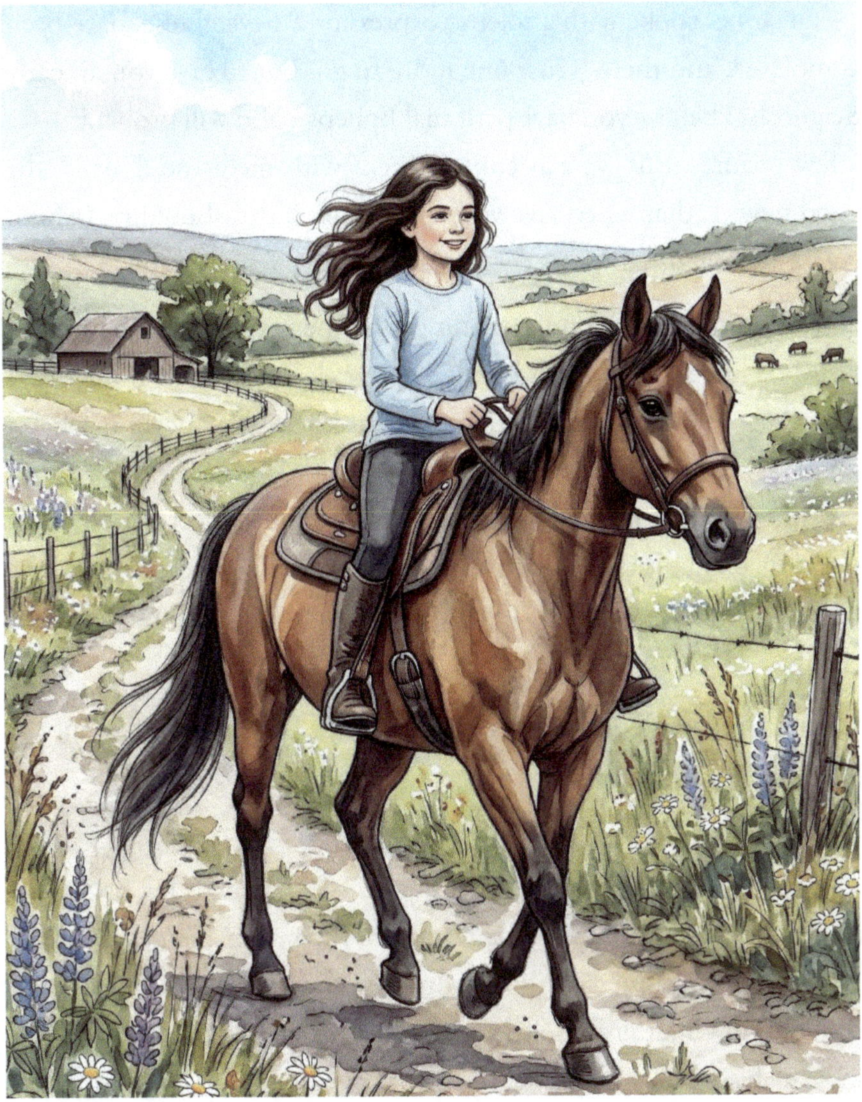

The next day, I stood up but immediately seemed to be dizzy again. The room tilted around me, and a wave of weakness passed through me. I sat back down on the bed and knew that something was not right with me. One hour later, Becky was on her way to the doctor with me, concern etched across her face.

Dr. Jones spoke with a solemn expression. "Several tests have been completed, and there is just one more to go. But to give you an early diagnosis, I believe you have petit mal Epilepsy. You will probably have a few seizures, but we can control them with medicine. Finally, the good news is that when five years have passed, this should be behind you. Petit mal usually lasts five years with just a few seizures."

I had a hard time understanding what he was saying. I had never heard of Epilepsy, and I had not had any seizures, at least none that I knew of. The words sounded strange and heavy, far beyond what a thirteen-year-old girl expected to hear in a doctor's office. He further explained that while there is no "recovery period", effects can include learning difficulties, behavioral changes, emotional challenges and potential injury from falls. I was given Tegretol to help me with the changes.

But Dr. Jones continued, explaining that I could still play sports, just not contact sports.

I thought to myself, *He did not say I couldn't ride Molly. I will not mention Molly to him.* At that thought, I felt some of my happiness return. *I am now thirteen. Just five more years of medicine, and I will be okay.* I continued with my dreams, most of them filled with thoughts of Chase and Molly, the two things that brought the most joy into my heart.

They drove most of the way in silence. I watched the fields pass outside the window, counting fence posts the way I always did when I needed to think.

Finally, I said, "Becky?"

"Yes, love?"

"Five years isn't that long, is it?"

Becky kept her eyes on the road, but her hand reached over and covered mine. "No," she said. "It is not. And you will not do a single day of it alone."

I turned back to the window. Outside, a horse was running alongside the fence line, mane lifted by the wind.

I watched it until it disappeared, and then I sat a little straighter.

Getting to fraternize with boys was a pleasure I looked forward to every day, especially when it came to Chase. His presence had begun to occupy more of my thoughts than I cared to admit, and even through the uncertainty of my diagnosis, the thought of seeing him still brought a quiet smile to my face.

CHAPTER TWO

There were several school events that occurred that gave me the opportunity to see Chase and, finally, to sneak in moments of holding hands when no one was looking. Those small touches, brief and secret, meant more to me than I could ever say.

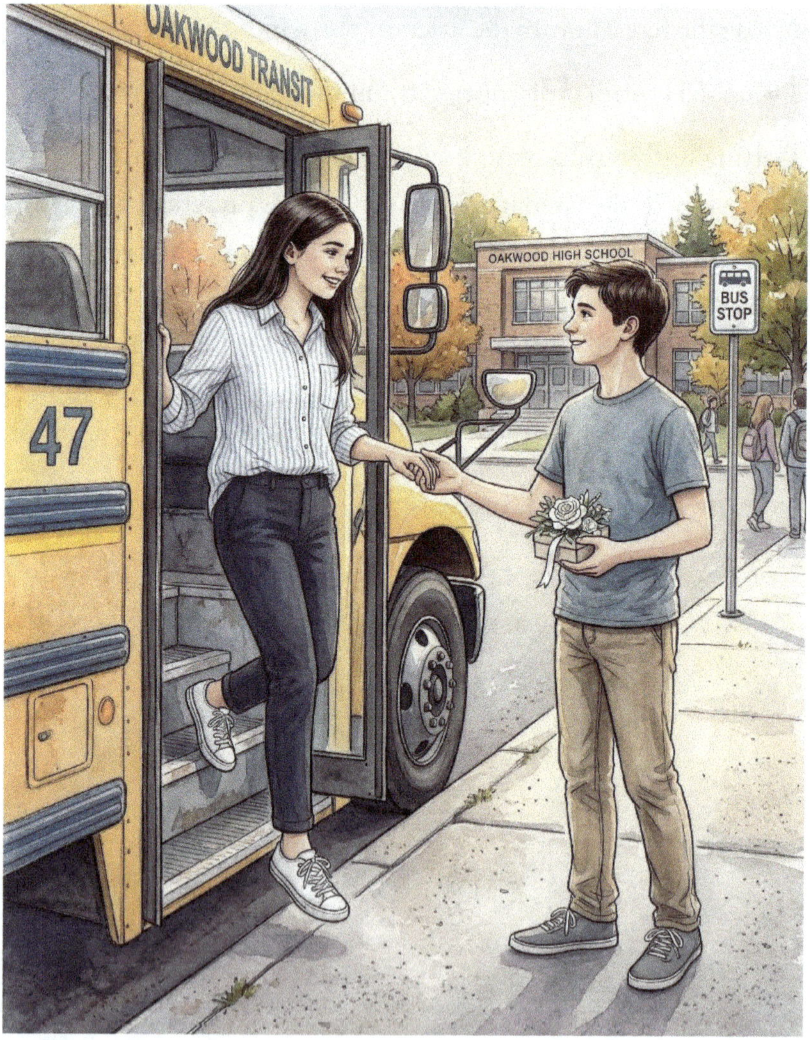

We girls at the orphanage were allowed to attend some of the activities, but not all of them. The Junior-Senior prom, however, was allowed. I was now sixteen, soon to be seventeen. I had joined the school choir and sometimes could stay after school to practice when the bus was available to take the late students home.

Becky took me shopping and found just the right prom dress, all violet, with scattered pearls on the bodice. I could hardly wait to wear it, to dance around, swirling the dress as I spun in front of the mirror. Finally, we found the shoes. Everything was perfect. *How can I be so lucky?* I thought. The only thing missing was Chase. If only I could ride with him to school, but rules had to be obeyed.

I could attend the prom and ride the bus to school and return, but Chase was not allowed to escort me in his car. Not yet.

Chase met me at the bus door, holding a corsage. He helped me down from the bus steps and carefully placed the lilac flowers on my arm. The color matched my dress perfectly. The fragrance was soft and unmistakable. *How did he know?* My heart swelled with joy, and for a moment I felt as if the entire evening had been made just for me.

"You look..." Chase started, then stopped, as if the right word had slipped just out of reach. "You look like you belong up on that stage."

I glanced down at the lilac flowers on my arm, then back up at him. "How did you know violet?"

He smiled, slow and a little shy. "I asked Becky."

I did not know what to say to that. The thought of Chase calling the orphanage, asking Becky, choosing carefully, it was almost more than I could hold. I laughed instead, softly, and he offered me his arm.

"Shall we?" he said.

I took it. "We shall," I replied, and we walked through the doors together as though it were the most natural thing in the world.

The bus would depart for home at 11:00 p.m. At 10:00, Chase held my hand and quietly led me out the side door near the restrooms, hoping no one saw us. The excitement of slipping away together sent a thrill through me, though deep inside I knew we were crossing a line. That rendezvous was the beginning of a situation that might not be easily solved.

The night air outside was cool and still, a sharp contrast to the warmth and noise of the gymnasium we had just left behind. Chase leaned against the brick wall, still holding my hand, and looked up at the sky.

"You're not scared?" he asked.

"A little," I admitted. "Are you?"

"Terrified," he said cheerfully, which made me laugh despite myself.

We sat on the low stone steps just around the corner, far enough from the doors to feel invisible. For a while, neither of us said anything. The distant sound of music drifted through the walls, muffled and dreamy.

"We should probably go back in," I said, after a time.

"Probably," Chase agreed. Neither of us moved.

I looked at him sideways. "You planned this, didn't you?"

He turned, eyes bright with something I could not quite name. "I just wanted five minutes where nobody was watching the clock but us."

I did not answer. I did not need to. The bus horn at eleven o'clock answered for me, and we ran.

***

At school, I was secretary to the Agriculture Department. The project for the year was to develop gardening guidelines for rural home buyers. I was instrumental in developing simply written guidelines for the young farmers. Procedures were already in place, but the class wanted to help the farmers in any way they could. We held fundraisers, selling vegetable seeds, and even assisted young farmers in planting gardens. This was something I truly enjoyed, partly because Chase was part of the group and partly because it reminded me of the work and life I had always known at the orphanage.

A trip was planned to take the school group to the next county to attend the Ag Convention. The excitement of traveling with classmates made the whole event feel special. At 9:00 p.m., when the seminar was finished, Chase and I chose that moment to disappear.

It was midnight before the girls rooming with me realized that I was not in my bed. At first, they thought perhaps I had gone to the restroom or had stepped out for water, but as the minutes passed, worry set in. The counselor was notified. A search began, and by morning, the two of us runaways were discovered sleeping in the back of the counselor's car.

The counselor, Mr. Holt, stood outside the car door with his arms crossed, looking more exhausted than angry.

"Tera. Chase." His voice was flat and even. "Do either of you have anything to say for yourselves?"

Chase sat up first, blinking in the early morning light. "Sir, it wasn't, we weren't doing anything wrong. We just fell asleep."

"You disappeared at nine o'clock at night without telling a single soul," Mr. Holt said. "Half the staff has been awake all night."

I looked at my hands. The shame of it was heavier than I had expected. "I'm sorry," I said quietly. "We didn't think about how it would look to everyone else."

Mr. Holt let out a long breath. "That," he said, "is precisely the problem."

No amount of explanation excused us.

Becky was concerned, not knowing exactly how to address this. Maybe this was part of the changes Dr. Jones spoke of, behavioral and emotional changes.

That evening, Becky sat across from me at the small desk in her office, the same bay window behind her where she had always done her thinking. She did not raise her voice. She did not need to.

"Do you understand why I'm worried?" she asked.

"Because I disappeared," I said.

"Because you didn't think," Becky said gently. "You've always been so careful, Tera. Thoughtful. And I need to know that girl is still in there, even when Chase is nearby."

I looked at her for a long moment. "She is," I said. "I promise she is."

Becky studied me the way she always did, as though she were reading something written just beneath the surface. Then she nodded, once, and reached across the desk and squeezed my hand.

"Good," she said. "Because I didn't raise a girl who loses herself."

I did not sleep well that night, but not from guilt alone. Her words stayed with me, turning over and over, the way only the truest things do.

I lost my secretary title. But we were happy, and no amount of chastising seemed to matter to us in that moment. Chase was given a failing grade, with no other penalty. All of this meant that I would see less of Chase. A quick kiss in the hallways was all that could now be expected. No other contact was allowed.

It was Chase who found me first, the morning after everything was settled. He fell into step beside me in the hallway between second and third period, his voice low.

"I'm sorry about your title," he said. "That's my fault."

"It's both our faults," I told him.

"Still." He paused at the bend in the corridor, where the hall split and we would each have to go a different way. He looked at me with that same steadiness he'd had since the very first bus ride. "It was worth it. Wasn't it?"

I thought of the cool night air, the muffled music through the gymnasium wall, the two of us sitting on those stone steps as if the rest of the world had agreed to wait.

"Yes," I said. "It was."

He smiled, and we went our separate ways down the hall.

But soon, school would be over, and to me, that thought carried both hope and uncertainty.

CHAPTER THREE

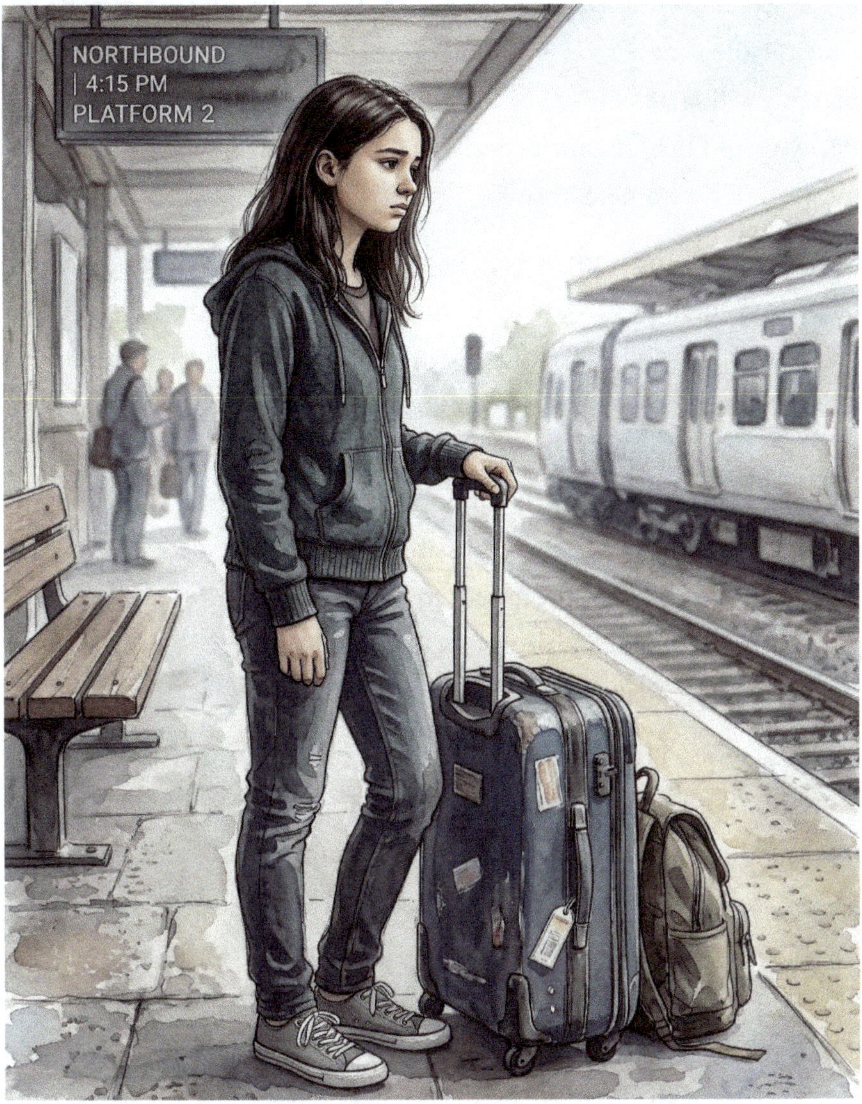

I graduated. At the age of eighteen, I could now leave the home I had grown up in. I was not sure what that would actually mean, or how life beyond the orphanage walls would truly feel. For so many years, every day had been guided by routine, familiar faces, and the quiet comfort of knowing exactly where I belonged. Now, everything ahead of me seemed wide open and uncertain. I would soon find out. Becky was still the one person I could count on to talk to, the one steady presence who had helped guide me through every stage of growing up. Becky would help me make decisions about a career and what it truly meant to leave home. She was my rock.

When I left the orphanage, I was granted $2,500.00 to begin a new life. All residents received an allowance when they left, something to help them start out on their own and take their first steps into adulthood. Even so, I knew it would not last forever. Decisions had to be made, and for the first time, those decisions belonged entirely to me. I had already begun to think of different options and different opportunities, though each possibility seemed both exciting and overwhelming. Becky promised to help search out opportunities, guiding me as I made my decisions and gently reminding me that I did not have to face it all alone.

First, a job. The allowance given to me would not last long. I had moved in with a graduate from the previous year, Penny. Penny had reached out to me, remembering how hard it had been when she herself had first left the orphanage and entered the world alone. I gladly accepted the offer. The kindness touched me deeply, and it gave me a sense of comfort to know someone understood exactly what I was feeling. I now had a place to live. Now I needed work.

Penny had called the week before graduation, her voice easy and warm in a way that immediately set me at ease.

"Tera, listen. I remember standing at that door with one bag and absolutely no idea what came next. You don't have to do that alone if you don't want to."

"I don't want to be a burden," I told her honestly.

"A burden," Penny repeated, and I could hear the smile in her voice. "Girl, you would be paying half the rent. That's not a burden, that's a blessing. Besides," she added, more softly, "it gets quiet out here. I could use the company."

I thought of the orphanage, always full of voices and motion, and tried to imagine silence as something that could press down on you rather than simply rest.

"Okay," I said. "Yes. Thank you, Penny."

"Don't thank me yet," she said cheerfully. "Wait until you see how small the bathroom is."

I laughed for the first time in days, and just like that, the future seemed a little less like a cliff edge and a little more like a road.

My love of horses gave me the perfect opportunity to apply at the next stable owner's ranch. The owner had advertised in the local paper for help. When the owner, Ms. Novel, met me, she immediately knew that I was a sharp, understanding person her ranch needed. There was something natural in the way I spoke about horses, a quiet confidence and affection that could not be taught. I could care for the horses as well as help with teaching the students who were learning to ride. I was quickly accepted among the other workers, and slowly I began to fit in with the other girls, finding a new rhythm to life outside the orphanage.

***

The following week, while feeding my favorite animals on earth, I saw Chase. He had graduated the year before and had left for college. Although we had written to each other, the letters had become fewer between his studies and my own preparations for graduation. At times, it had seemed as though he had found other interests, but my heart still leaned toward him. Even with time and distance between us, something inside me had never truly let go.

What is he doing here? I thought, my heart suddenly racing.

Chase spotted me, and upon seeing me, ran toward me, grabbing hold of me and swinging me around and around. Laughter burst from both of us as if no time at all had passed. It was as though time had stood still for us, preserving every memory and every feeling exactly where it had been left.

"What are you doing here?" I asked, breathless with surprise and happiness.

He answered, "Ms. Novel is my aunt. I am just visiting, but I think my visiting just got extended."

He remembered. He remembered the sweet young girl who had stolen his heart. And I remembered my first kiss from this handsome boy, a memory that had remained tucked safely in my heart all these years.

When the laughter finally settled, we leaned side by side against the fence the way we used to do, letting the quiet find us.

"I wasn't sure you'd still be here," Chase said, his voice lower now, stripped of the giddiness.

"I wasn't sure you'd still come looking," I answered.

He turned to look at me, squinting a little against the afternoon light. “I always come looking. You should know that by now.”

I kept my eyes on the horses moving in the far pasture, not trusting my face to stay still. “Letters got short,” I said.

“I know.” He was quiet for a moment. “Studying got hard. I got afraid I’d run out of things to say and you’d stop writing back.”

“Chase,” I said, turning to him at last, “I would have written back if you’d sent me a grocery list.”

He laughed, startled, and some of the tension between us dissolved into the afternoon air. We stood there a while longer, side by side, not needing to say anything more.

By the end of the day, I was so excited about seeing Chase again that I might have forgotten to finish my chores, but Chase pitched in and helped. Together we moved easily through the work, laughing and talking as though we had never been apart. That left us a couple of hours at the end of the day to sit and talk, catching up on everything life had brought since we last truly shared time together.

Chase followed me home that day. He never left.

Our relationship was kept secret for a couple of months, but it was not long before the town folks knew that we were a “budding” couple. In a town that noticed everything, our growing closeness quickly became something whispered about with warm smiles and knowing glances.

***

Chase was to return back to college in one more month. He simply could not bear the thought of going and leaving me behind again.

"What do we tell your aunt?" I inquired, my voice carrying both hope and uncertainty.

Chase answered, not entirely sure of himself, but firm in what he wanted. "We will share my apartment while I finish. I have one more year, and then we can get married. My degree in financing will help me get a good job, hopefully close to home," he said.

His aunt did not think it was a good idea for him to try to finish school and support a wife at the same time. She spoke with the wisdom of someone who had seen how difficult life could become when love had to compete with responsibility. So, with some persuasion, I remained behind, though it was not an easy decision for either of us.

Christmas came around, and Chase came home again, this time to hear my news.

"I am going to have a baby!" I blurted out as soon as he stepped out of the truck. The words rushed out of me, unable to be held back any longer. I was excited, but scared too. This had not been part of our plans, but now it had become a new plan, one that would shape both of our lives.

Chase stood still for a second or two, the surprise settling over him, and then he recovered enough to pick me up and swing me around the way he used to do. For a moment, neither of us could speak. The reality of what I had said hung between us, filled with fear, joy, and the weight of everything still ahead.

Finally, after spending time pondering, making choices, and weighing decisions, we decided to leave me with his aunt. He would return to school and finish in five months. He would be home in time to be with me when the baby arrived. If he applied himself more, he could finish his classes a month early, come home, and then just go back to graduate. We did not want to part again, but we both believed this would be best. Time seemed to creep by, each day moving slower than the last, as I waited for the day I would once again be with Chase and for the new addition to my life to arrive.

***

Chase made it home with three weeks to spare. He was there the morning the contractions started, pacing the small kitchen while I sat at the table, breathing through each wave with my eyes fixed on a point just above the windowsill.

"Shouldn't we go?" he asked, for what felt like the fourth time.

"Not yet," I said.

"How do you know?"

I looked at him over my shoulder. "Because I'll tell you when."

He sat down across from me, pressed his hands flat on the table, and nodded as though I had said something very sensible. "Okay," he said. "Okay." Then, a moment later: "Shouldn't we..."

"Chase."

"Right. Sorry."

By the time we reached the hospital, the world had narrowed down to one room and one purpose, and Chase held my hand so tightly I was not sure which of us was holding the other up. When it was over and the nurse placed the baby in his arms for the first time, something in Chase's face changed completely. Every worry, every restless plan, every uncertain future, all of it went quiet at once.

"He looks like you," Chase said softly.

"He's bald," I replied, my voice gone thin with exhaustion and laughter at the same time.

"Beautifully bald." Chase looked up at me, his eyes bright. "Chason," he said, as though confirming the name to himself and to the room and to every piece of the future all at once. "That's who you are."

Chason was born the day after graduation. Weighing just a little over seven pounds, he was perfect, arriving in what we felt was perfect timing. Chase and I were so delighted to be new parents, to hold our little baby boy and begin making dreams with him. I had never been happier than I was then. Holding him in my arms, I felt a kind of love I had never known before, deeper than words and stronger than anything I had ever imagined.

We moved in together in the next town over from the ranch. I got another job working at the veterinary hospital, caring for large animals. I loved the horses and the other large animals that were sometimes hospitalized. Being near them gave me comfort and reminded me of the part of myself that had always been strongest. The wedding was on hold until money was no longer so scarce. Chason was being cared for by Becky and the girls at the orphanage. He was in good hands, especially with me sometimes working late to accommodate the injured animals that needed extra attention and care. Even so, there were nights when exhaustion settled over me, and I would think, *if only Chase was here more.*

***

Chase graduated from college. Our town was a small town, and to do the job he truly wanted, he would need to move to where jobs were available. After two months of sending out resumes and going for interviews, he was becoming disillusioned. Each rejection seemed to weigh more heavily on him than the one before. He felt as though he were up against a wall and did not know what would be best for our little family. The dreams that once felt so close now seemed just out of reach, and the pressure of providing for me and Chason pressed heavily on his heart.

He had been thinking more every day about what to do and where to go to find work. He did not want to live anywhere else. The thought of leaving the town, the ranch, and the life we had begun to build together weighed heavily on him. Without discussing the decision with his aunt or with me, he made a choice. It was hard to understand why he did not discuss the options with me. Chase did not want to explain himself. Being unable to provide a steady income and not wanting to live anywhere else, this seemed like the only answer. He spent many nights sleepless, wanting to tell me what he was going to do, but he could not bear the thought of seeing disappointment in my face.

He told me on a Tuesday evening, after supper, when Chason was already asleep and the house had gone quiet. I knew something was coming. He had been careful with me for days in the way people are when they are carrying something they have not yet put down.

"There is something I need to tell you," he said. He was sitting across from me at the kitchen table, turning his coffee cup slowly in his hands.

"Then tell me," I said.

He looked up. "I joined the Army."

The words landed in the quiet of the room and just stayed there. I did not speak right away. I counted three full breaths before I could find anything to say that was not made entirely of fear.

"When?"

"Two weeks ago. I'm leaving in two weeks."

"Chase." My voice came out smaller than I intended. "You didn't tell me. You didn't even ask me."

"I know." He set the cup down. "I couldn't. Every time I tried, I looked at you and I just, I couldn't bear for you to look at me the way you're looking at me right now."

"How am I looking at you?"

"Like I'm leaving," he said quietly.

I pressed my hands flat on the table, the way he used to do when he was trying to hold himself steady. "Will you come back?"

"Always," he said. The word was immediate and sure, the most certain thing he had said all evening. "I will always come back to you and Chason. I just need to find a way to deserve coming back."

I did not say anything more that night. But I reached across the table and held his hand, and we sat that way for a long time, the sleeping baby in the next room and the uncertain road ahead of us, and neither of us let go.

Chase went to the local Army recruiter. The final decision was made with the help of the sergeant at the desk. He joined the Army. With his degree, he would be entering as a Second Lieutenant, with very good pay and very good benefits. Chase and I would have those benefits as well. For the first time in weeks, he felt as though he had found a way forward, a path that would allow him to provide for our family. Now he had to face me and his aunt.

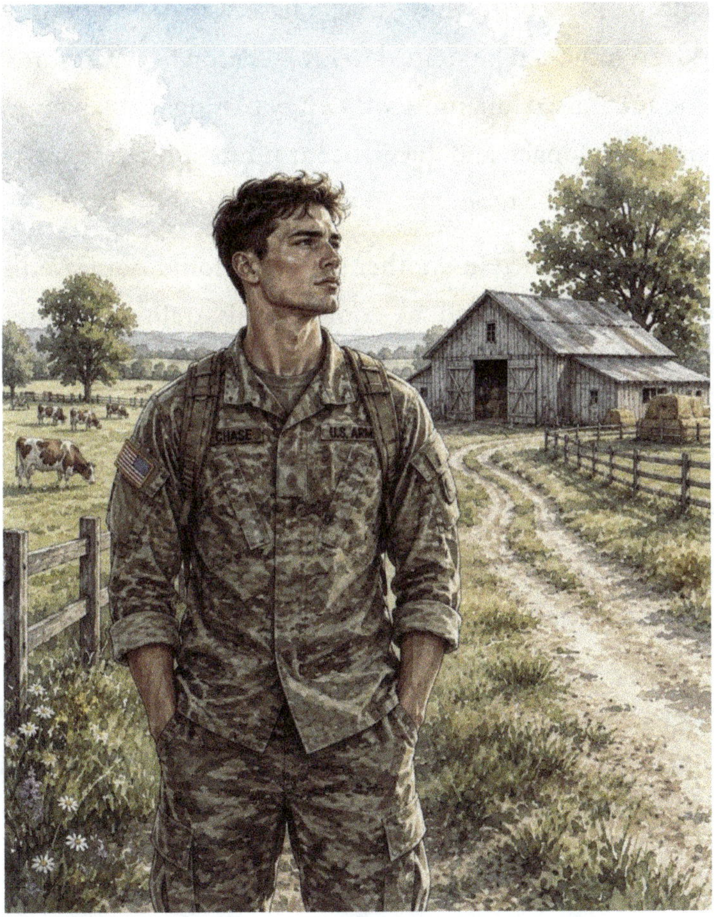

Two weeks later, Chase was leaving. I, baby Chason, and his aunt all went to the airport to say our goodbyes. The moment felt heavier than any of us had expected. Not knowing when we might see him again, we left feeling very sad, burdened by the uncertainty of what tomorrow might bring. I held Chason close, trying to memorize the sight of Chase standing there, as if holding onto the image might somehow make the separation easier.

It was not long before I became disillusioned with the plans for a wedding. The distance, the waiting, and the uncertainty began to wear on my heart. I began to think that Chase was not anxious to be a husband, even though he seemed to love Chason beyond words. I was lonesome and missed him more with every passing moment away from him. Nights felt longer, and the silence around me often seemed louder than the voices in the room.

Chase was stationed in another state and could not leave the base for three months. He had to complete his training before being assigned. After his training, Chase got his orders to report to Germany in thirty days. There would be no wedding until he returned. After receiving his orders to leave, Chase called me to let me know he would be in Atlanta to fly out and wanted to see me before leaving.

I fearfully decided to go see him. Questions raced through my mind, each one more painful than the last. *Is he calling me to cancel our wedding plans? He had not given me a ring yet. Maybe he wants to solidify our wedding plans. Does he still want to get married? Does he want to be a father to Chason?* My heart pounded, and my hands grew cold with anxiety. But I had to know.

I hurriedly made plans to go to the airport to tell him goodbye. His aunt and I, along with Chason, left the following day for Atlanta. I was so excited to see him, but also deeply sad because it might be a long time before seeing him again, if he still wanted me in his life. Fear shook me to my bones.

I spotted Chase as soon as I entered the airport. He had been waiting, hoping with all his heart that I would come. The moment our eyes met, all the fear and distance of the past months seemed to collapse into that single instant. Chase ran to me and grabbed Chason and me at the same time, pulling us close as if he never wanted to let go again.

He began to whisper, "I love you. I can hardly wait for you to be my wife."

I could hardly believe he had said that. My heart skipped a beat, and for a moment the noise of the airport seemed to disappear around me. A second or two later, I responded with a happy softness in my voice, though the emotion rising in my chest nearly stole my breath away. I could not find the words I wanted to say, so instead I simply held on to him as tightly as I could, pouring everything I felt into that embrace.

Soon, the plane was ready to take on the passengers. Chase held on to my hand tightly as we walked to the gate. He kept looking at me as though he were trying to sear my face into his mind, memorizing every detail before he had to leave again. Then the moment came, and he had to go. I waved goodbye tearfully with Chason. *Two years is a long time to be away,* I thought, and I wondered if he was thinking the same thing.

For the next six months, letters flew back and forth between us. Those letters became a lifeline, filled with small details, reassurances, and promises of the future. He talked of coming home on leave, but that date was unknown even to him. To help pass the time, he began going with his Army buddies to the local pub. The soldiers began to talk about being transferred to Saudi Arabia. It seemed that trouble was brewing there, and the military was going to be sent to protect the American Embassy.

We both started to realize that time had given us space to grow a little older and maybe a little wiser. The warm, cuddly feelings were no longer as frequent as they once had been. His telephone calls were becoming less and less. Each missed call and each longer silence left a mark on my heart. I slowly began to accept that I was on my own now and would have to make things work for myself and for Chason. Sadly, I noticed that my feelings were changing.

***

There was an evening in early November when I sat at the kitchen table after Chason had fallen asleep, a letter half-written in front of me and the pen set to one side. I had been staring at the same sentence for twenty minutes.

Penny came in from her shift and set her keys on the counter. She looked at the letter, then at me.

“Haven’t sent that one yet?” she said, without judgment.

“I don’t know what to say anymore,” I admitted.

Penny pulled out the chair across from me and sat down slowly, the way she did when she was not in a hurry to be anywhere else. “What do you want to say?”

I looked at the letter. "I want to say that Chason said a new word today. I want to say that the bay mare at the clinic finally let me close without shying. I want to say I'm proud of him and I'm waiting." I paused. "But I also want to say that waiting is getting harder than I thought it would be, and I don't know if writing that is fair to him or honest or just selfish."

Penny was quiet for a moment. Then she said, "Write the first part. The baby, the horse. Save the second part for when he's standing in front of you and can answer it."

It was good advice. I picked up the pen.

But the second part did not wait. It grew quietly, the way things do when they are not spoken, taking up more room with every week that passed and every call that came later than expected, or not at all.

I noticed a cowboy who would come into the clinic to pick up medicine for his horse. At first, it was only a brief conversation, but soon those small exchanges became something more familiar. We began to talk. He told me about his ranch and about his horses, speaking with the same kind of affection I had always carried for them. I told him of my engagement to Chase and of my little boy, Chason. He did not seem to comprehend the message that I was already involved in a relationship. Or perhaps he understood perfectly and simply did not care.

He was there, and he wanted me.

Several days went by, and he consistently called me and asked me out. I was listening.

He was not.

I was so excited about meeting a cowboy that I called my best friend, Penny, and shared the story with her.

"Penny, I met a cowboy. I have always wanted a cowboy with lots of horses who loves to ride, and I think I will say yes to seeing him. Chase is gone, and he is ignoring plans for a wedding. Maybe I should reconsider my options, too."

My voice carried a mixture of excitement, confusion, and guilt, as if I were speaking thoughts aloud that I had only just begun to admit.

"Penny, every time I see him, I do not want to leave. I told Chase about him last night. His only concern was for Chason. He looked worried about losing me, but also seemed to be okay with my decision. Chase told me of someone he had met."

The words hung heavily in the air.

I was now alone.

Not just physically, but emotionally as well. The future I had once imagined with Chase no longer seemed certain, and the life I had carefully held together was beginning to shift beneath my feet.

THE SET-UP

After six weeks of seeing Cowboy Tom, nicknamed Bubba, I agreed to marry him. He convinced me that he could support me and Chason in a better style, with a better home and a better life. So, sight unseen as to his living arrangements or to his style of living, I agreed to marry him. There was no time to discuss it with friends. He planned the wedding for just two weeks away, leaving no real time to think through my decision. He pressured me with love notes, with promises, and, most of all, with the promise of living on a beautiful ranch with lots of horses. To me, those words touched the deepest part of the dreams I had carried since childhood.

"Penny, he wants me to wear red when we get married. I have a beautiful white dress I found while shopping for a wedding with Chase. I want to walk down the aisle in white, but he wants me to wear red." I paused, trying to convince myself as much as Penny. Then I added softly, almost as if talking myself into it, "That is okay. I will wear red."

Penny set down her coffee cup slowly. "He wants you to wear red."

"It's just a color."

"Tera, you have a white dress. A beautiful one. You've had it for years. You picked it out yourself."

"I know." I looked at my hands. "But it's important to him. He has a thing about it."

"What kind of thing?"

I did not have a good answer for that. I had asked him once, lightly, and he had turned it into a conversation about how much he loved red on me, how it suited me, how he had always imagined this. He had a way of making his preferences sound like compliments. By the end of it, I had almost believed that wearing red had been my idea.

"It's fine, Penny," I said, with more certainty than I felt. "It's just a dress."

Penny looked at me the way she sometimes did, as though she could see something I was choosing not to.

"Since you and I are going to Laughlin, Nevada, to see your cousin, we could get married there. He wants to get married as soon as possible. Let's make arrangements to be there for December 15th," I continued.

The future planning started immediately, and to me it felt like security after a childhood of uncertainty. The quick pace of it all gave me something solid to hold on to, or at least that was what I wanted to believe. I made plans for the girls I knew from the orphanage to be there with me. The orphanage had been my life. Everyone important to me had lived there with me all my life. They would attend. Just two weeks to plan it all. Penny reminded me that I had only known him for less than two months.

"Are you sure about this, Tera?" Penny asked. "After all, none of your friends have met him, have talked with him, nor even been invited out to celebrate with you!"

I turned to face her. I had been half-expecting this, and I had already rehearsed the answer somewhere in the back of my mind.

"I know it's fast," I said. "But I know how I feel. And he is good to me, Penny. He is kind and attentive and he makes me feel like I matter. You know how long it's been since someone made me feel like that."

"I do know," Penny said carefully. "That's what worries me. When someone comes along at exactly the right moment and says exactly the right things, Tera, sometimes that's real. But sometimes it's just someone who has learned how to read a person."

"He's not like that."

"How do you know? You've known him six weeks."

The room went quiet. I could feel the shape of the argument, the edge of it, and I did not want to step any closer. I reached over and took Penny's hand instead.

"Come with me," I said. "Please. I need you there. If you are standing beside me, then at least I know someone who loves me is in the room."

Penny looked at me for a long moment. Then she closed her eyes briefly and let out a slow breath.

"Of course I'll be there," she said quietly. "I'm always going to be there."

I stood silently for a moment more, my mind still clouded with something I could not quite name. Somewhere deep inside, doubt had begun to stir, yet I pushed forward, unwilling to slow down long enough to face what that doubt might mean.

***

Finally, it was time for the wedding. I walked down the aisle wearing red. I had a beautiful white gown hanging in my closet, the one I had bought when I was engaged to Chase. *What will I do with the white dress?* I pondered. The thought lingered in the back of my mind like a quiet ache. But to fulfill his unusual request, I wore a red dress.

None of his family attended. Not one person.

One of my orphanage friends, standing just to my left before the ceremony began, leaned toward me and said in a low voice, "Tera, where is his family?"

I kept my eyes forward. "He said they couldn't make the trip."

"All of them?"

I did not answer that. I adjusted the sash on my red dress and reminded myself to smile. There would be time to ask him about it later, I told myself. There was a reasonable explanation. There always was.

What I could not explain away so easily was the feeling that crept over me when I realized there was not a single face in that room who was there for him. Every person standing in that space had come for me.

I wondered why, but I did not question it. My instincts tried to warn me several times during this period, but I pushed those feelings away because they did not match the fairy-tale story unfolding around me. I wanted so badly to believe in the life he had promised me that I ignored the unease rising inside. We had two nights in Vegas for our honeymoon, then went back to our home.

What I did not know about Tom was that he already had two children by two different women and was paying child support for both of them. He was also twelve years older than I was. He was a jealous, revengeful, unkind, inconsiderate, selfish person, as I would soon find out. At the time, none of this was visible to me. It all became clear only to those looking in from the outside. He presented himself to his family as a genuine person, but those who knew him outside of that circle recognized the imbalance he displayed when angry or jealous. The warning signs were there, hidden beneath charm and promises. But again, I did not know.

He was still on his best behavior.

Still believing whatever lie he told, I proceeded with the relationship. He always seemed to know the right words to say at the right time, and my mind began to hear security in his voice, even when that was never truly his intention. To me, his words sounded like stability, protection, and the promise of a future I had longed for all my life. I had been raised around honest, faithful women, women whose words and actions matched, so this kind of behavior was unknown to me. I did not recognize it for what it was.

He was not a patient man. However, he worked in a town one hundred and fifty miles away. Still, he tried to come home every night for the first two or three months. It was not because he missed me, but because he did not trust. He had a mobile trailer at his job, so he had a place to stay there, yet he refused to remain away. I encouraged him to stay at the job during the week and just come home on weekends. I thought it would be easier on him and better for our life together. Instead, he would call me as many as sixty-three times in one day, depending on his dysfunctional mood. The constant ringing became a shadow over every hour of my day. I found it hard to focus at work, always having to answer the phone, always wondering what mood would be waiting for me on the other end of the line.

The calls followed a pattern I came to dread. My phone would ring before I had finished my first cup of coffee.

"What are you doing?"

"Getting ready for work," I said.

"Who's there?"

I paused. "No one. It's seven in the morning, Tom."

"I heard a voice."

"That was the television."

A silence followed, the kind that was not empty but full, pressing.

"Turn it off."

"I need the news on while I get dressed."

"Turn it off." His voice had not risen, which somehow made it worse. The flat, even tone of it carried more weight than shouting would have.

I turned off the television.

The call lasted another twenty minutes. When I finally reached work, I was already twelve minutes late and already bracing for the next ring. By lunch, my phone had logged eleven missed calls. By three o'clock, nineteen. By the time I drove home with Chason in the back seat, I had stopped counting.

"Mommy, why does the phone ring so much?" Chason asked from the back seat.

I looked at him in the rearview mirror. "It's just Papa checking in," I said.

Chason looked out the window. He did not say anything else. He had already learned when not to ask questions.

Eventually, I lost my job because of the phone calls. I had been warned several times by my employer to stop the interruptions, but I could not make him stop. The pressure from home had begun to spill into every part of my life. I was told that I could return in the future when my situation changed.

My supervisor, Mrs. Aldaine, had been patient with me longer than most would have been. She called me into her office on a Tuesday afternoon, closed the door quietly, and sat down across from me with the look of someone who had rehearsed what she was about to say.

"Tera, I like you. You are good at this job and you are good with the children. You know that."

"Yes, ma'am."

"But the phone calls cannot continue. I have spoken to you about this three times now. The other staff are covering for you while you step out, and it isn't fair to them, and it isn't sustainable for this classroom." She folded her hands on the desk. "Is everything alright at home?"

I felt heat rise in my face. "Yes. He just... he worries. It's new. He'll settle down."

Mrs. Aldaine looked at me the way Penny sometimes looked at me, as though she could see past the answer I had given to the one I had not.

"I hope so," she said gently. "Because if it continues, I won't have a choice. And I don't want to lose you."

I thanked her and went back to the classroom. That evening, Tom called forty-one times.

The following week, I was let go.

Rather than look for another job right away, I decided to take care of my friend's two children while she worked, and Chason would at least have playmates. For a while, that brought some comfort into the house. The sound of children playing softened the tension that had begun to settle around my life. Still, he continued to call. I often wondered how he could possibly find time away from his job to continue calling me so often. Then I found out that his father was his boss.

THE CRUELTY OF WORDS

Trouble started brewing. Unknown to me, he had his mail delivered to his parents' home, which included the cell phone bill. From the very beginning, he would question me about whom I was calling, why I was calling, and wanted to know the nature of every conversation. What had once seemed like concern now began to feel like something darker. He started imagining that any telephone call from or to a male indicated an outside intimate relationship. He had gone far beyond being reasonable. He was paranoid and controlling. I would cry, wondering if he would ever begin to trust me and whether we would ever live a pleasant life that did not include this constant suspicion and his paranoid disposition.

I was appalled at such insinuations. The accusations cut deeply because they were so far removed from the truth and from the kind of life I had believed marriage would be. He was checking the cell phone calls on a daily basis, then calling me up to question me about whom I had called and why. Each conversation felt less like a marriage and more like an interrogation.

The interrogations followed no particular schedule, which was part of what made them so exhausting. He could call at eight in the morning or ten at night, and the tone was always the same: measured, cold, and certain.

"There's a number on here I don't recognize."

I set down what I was doing. "Which one?"

He read out a number.

"That's the school," I said. "I called about Chason's field trip form."

Silence.

"Tom, it's the school."

"How do I know that?"

I pressed my free hand flat against the counter to keep myself steady. "Because I'm telling you. You can call them yourself and ask."

"Maybe I will."

He did not. He never did. The point was never to verify anything. The point was to make me feel that I owed him an explanation for every hour I breathed.

I began to have flashbacks of being under someone else's control, of feeling as though my life no longer belonged to me. *Where was the loving partnership of marriage?* I kept asking myself. My instincts tried to warn me several times during this period, but I pushed those feelings away because they did not match the fairy-tale story I had wanted so desperately to believe in. Those moments of unease got buried under the romantic gestures and declarations of love because I wanted so badly for this to be real. Yet, somewhere inside, the truth was beginning to press harder against my heart.

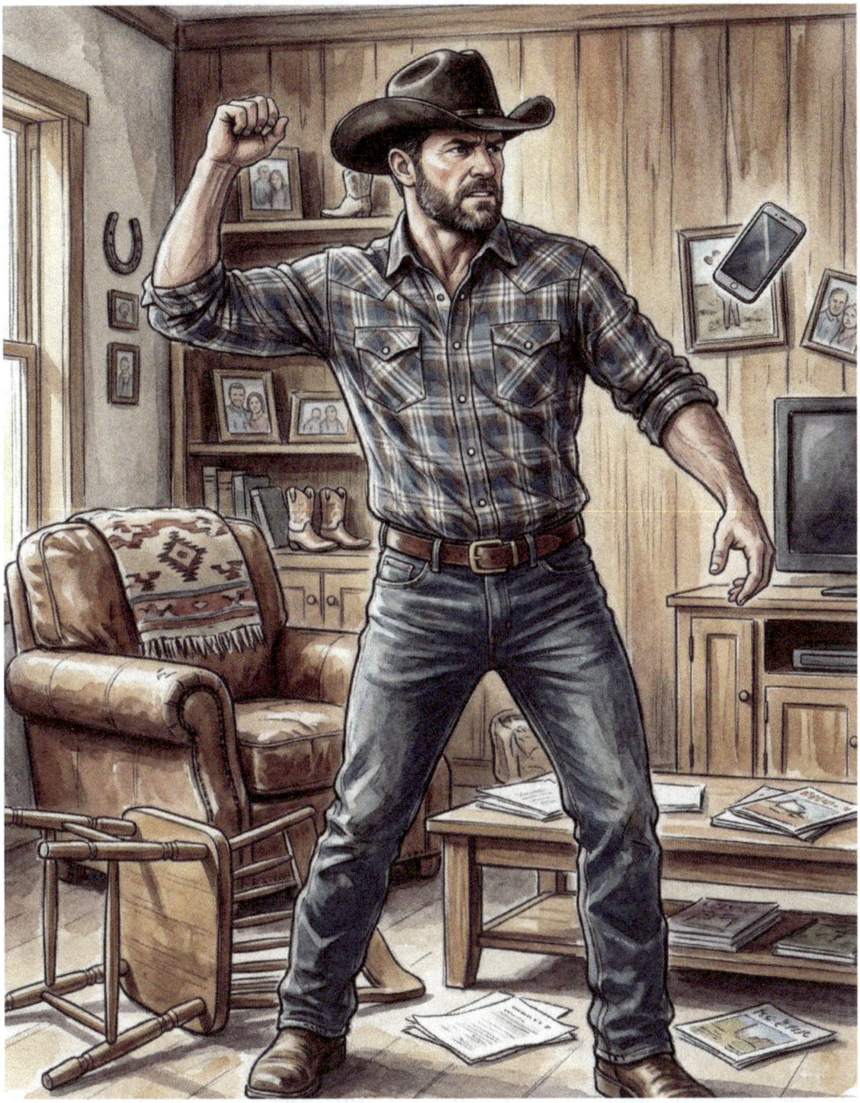

Doubts built up on some days. When I gave him answers that he did not like, he would take my phone and throw it against the wall. Breaking my new phones three times had cost him about a thousand dollars in replacements. So, he went from throwing phones to hitting his large television screen and breaking it. That left me without anything to watch while he was at work. Each outburst left me shaken, the sound of glass cracking and objects breaking lingering in my mind long after the moment had passed. I would threaten to leave each time this occurred, but he was a convincing sweet talker and could always get me to come around to his way of thinking. Being twelve years older, he often filled the role of a father, something I had never experienced. That stirred mixed feelings in me, feelings I did not fully understand, but I brushed them aside. He continued with his controlling ways, regardless of my growing feelings of concern.

I put my foot down when it came to talking to Chason's father. Chason deserved a dad who cared, and I was determined to keep him informed.

Bubba Tom would just have to live with that.

I had never been treated so disrespectfully in all my years at the orphanage. The women there had raised me with kindness, firmness, and dignity, and this life felt so far from the values I had grown up with. I was not sure what I should do or whom I should go to for help, and fear of embarrassment kept me silent. Part of me still hoped things would change, that the loving words he offered afterward meant something real.

Once he felt secure that I was hooked, the behavior started to change slowly. The constant texting became sporadic, the compliments turned into gentle criticisms, and the focused attention was redirected toward other things. By then, I was already trying to figure out how to get back to those magical early days instead of recognizing that they had never been real in the first place. I found myself replaying his earlier words in my mind, wondering what I had done differently, as if somehow, I could return them to what I had once believed was love.

I still had not gone to his ranch. He said he did not have time with all the traveling for his job. He told me the ranch was another hour away, but we would go soon. I started to wonder, *who is caring for the ranch and the horses?* The question lingered in my thoughts more and more often. We continued to live in my rental home, while the life he had promised remained something I had only ever seen in words.

I started noticing small things that just did not feel quite right, but I would dismiss them because everything else was supposed to feel so wonderful. He would get slightly irritated when I wanted to spend time with friends from the orphanage. Then he would bring me flowers and tell me he loved me so much that he wanted all of my time. At first, those words sounded romantic, almost flattering. But slowly, I began to sense something else beneath them. He was testing my boundaries and measuring my responses, seeing how much manipulation I would accept when it was wrapped in declarations of love.

Each day, the unease inside me grew a little stronger, though I still fought against naming it for what it truly was.

OUTRAGEOUS BEHAVIOR

One of the promises he made when working to convince me to leave Chase and marry him was that he would get me a car that would be safe for Chason to ride in. The vehicle I had been driving belonged to Becky and had been gifted to me until she was ready to get another vehicle.

Four months into the marriage, we went car shopping. We found a Hummer H3 that we both liked very well. To me, it felt like one more sign that perhaps the life he had promised was finally becoming real. We offered the dealership a deal with $3,000.00 down, signed the contract, and drove off. I could hardly believe it. I would ask him every hour, "Is this really mine?"

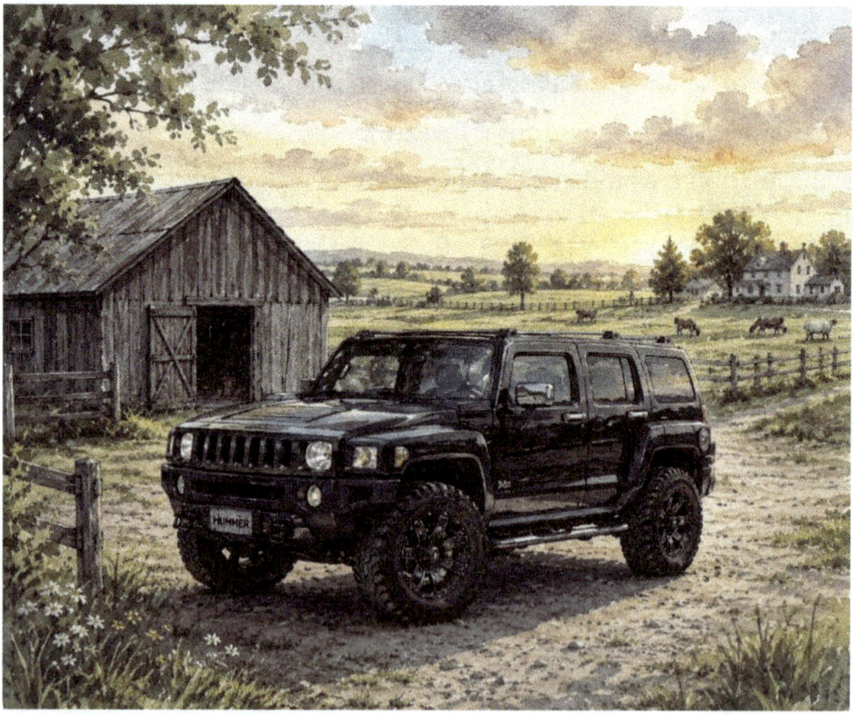

He would assure me that the vehicle was mine.

In those moments, he made me feel like the center of his universe. He wanted to become the standard against which I would measure all future relationships, creating an intensity that felt like devotion but was built on control. At the time, I could not yet see the difference.

That evening, I called Penny, barely able to sit still.

"Penny, he bought me a Hummer. A Hummer H3. I keep touching the steering wheel because I can't believe it's real."

Penny laughed. "A Hummer? Tera..."

"I know. I know. But it's mine. He said it's mine."

There was a brief pause. "Are you happy?" Penny asked.

"I am," I said. And in that moment, I was. I held onto that feeling through the night.

The following morning, Tom called.

"Take the car back," he said. "I need the money to pay taxes."

The words did not register at first. "What?"

"Take it back to the dealership today." His voice was flat, the way it always was when the decision had already been made and the conversation was just a formality.

I sat down on the edge of the bed. I had told everyone. I had posted it. I had called Penny. I had already begun to think of it as mine in the small, private way that made it real.

When I called Penny back, I did not have to say much.

"He's taking it back," I said.

There was a silence on Penny's end that said everything she was choosing not to say. Then, carefully: "Do you need me to come over?"

"No," I said. "I'm okay."

I was not okay. But I had already begun the work of convincing myself that I was.

This was not true. Money was not needed for taxes.

The sudden shift left me stunned and deeply unsettled. What had felt like a gift and a gesture of care now seemed like another way to keep me emotionally off balance. It made me feel trapped in the relationship, unsure of what was real and what was simply another one of his manipulations. I was beginning to think that I did not have the ability to recognize genuine love from possessive, controlling love. My mind could not separate the two feelings.

I had already posted on social media and called all my friends to tell them that he had bought me a car.

None of this made sense.

I called the dealership and asked if they would take the Pontiac that Becky had given me in exchange and return the money. They agreed.

However, Tom had already called the salesperson with such a demanding and aggressive attitude that it caused them to refuse to make the exchange. The salesperson said, "It is not returnable."

Once Tom was defeated on that issue, he again told me the vehicle was mine and reassured me that he would not take it from me.

The cycle was becoming painfully familiar. First, the gift. Then the threat of taking it away. Then the sweet reassurance.

Arguments were occurring more often now. He still insisted on driving home every night. He did not trust that I was home alone. In his mind, he did not know what I might be doing.

Now I had a beautiful vehicle to ride around in and, in his eyes, attract attention.

This he could not handle.

I asked that he stay at his job site during the week, not only to save the gas money but also for safety in driving such a long distance every day. The constant travel, the constant calls, and the constant suspicion were beginning to wear on me.

He was becoming more controlling every day.

I, in turn, became more resistant to his behavior.

Even the way he treated others began to disturb me. He would deny his daughter from his first marriage her requests to visit on the weekends. He did not want his daughter to come because, as he coldly put it, "she was in the way of his good time."

Those words stayed with me.

For the first time, I began to see more clearly that the cruelty I had been experiencing was not occasional anger but part of who he truly was.

CONTROLLED BEHAVIOR

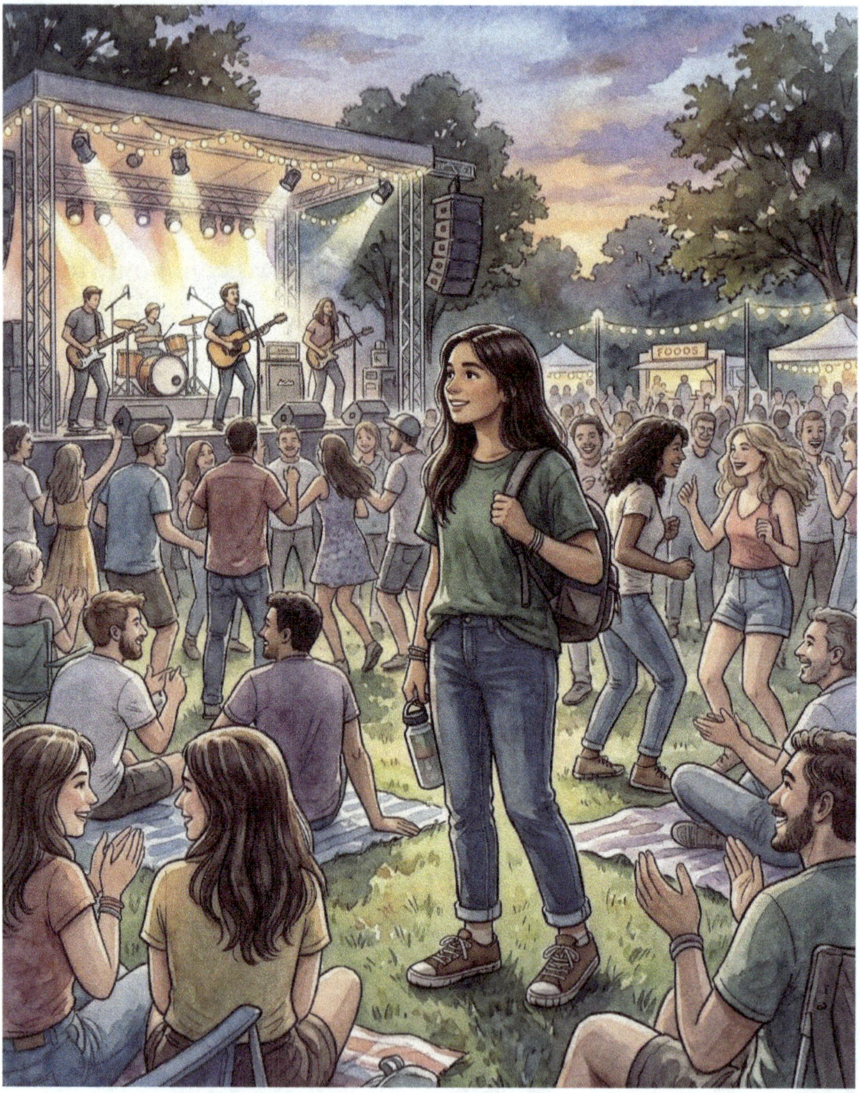

Another month went by, and Tom bought tickets to an outdoor concert featuring Gary Allan. I was so excited that we were going. For a moment, it felt like one of the happier times I had once imagined marriage would bring.

I dressed carefully that evening, pulling on my cowboy boots with the kind of quiet excitement I had not felt in a while. When I came into the living room, Tom looked at me for a moment.

"You look good," he said.

It was such a simple thing to say. But I held onto it.

"Thank you." I turned once, letting the hem of my shirt catch the light. "I've been looking forward to this all week."

"Gary Allan puts on a real show," he said, and for a moment he seemed easy and relaxed, the version of him I still sometimes caught glimpses of. "You'll love it."

I wanted to love it. I wanted that evening to be the kind of evening married people were supposed to have, music and open air and laughter, and maybe a small reminder of why I had said yes in the first place.

For a while, standing in the crowd with the music swelling around us, it almost was.

I was tiny, so Tom lifted me up onto his shoulders so I could see the show better. The heels of my boots dug into his chest as I tried to stay balanced on his shoulders. They left marks on his chest, but he did not complain.

A woman standing behind us at the concert started complaining that I was blocking her view while sitting on his shoulders. The woman was ignored. Tom made a remark to her, and she was offended by what he said, so she reached forward and put gum in my hair. Before I could even react, Tom turned around and said something again to the woman, and she punched him on the left temple, causing it to swell.

"Say that again, and I will punch you again!" she yelled.

I quickly climbed down and hurried to get ice to put on his eye. The evening had shifted so quickly from excitement to chaos that I hardly had time to process it. Tom had already had several beers, so I drove us home.

Once we were home, I got into the shower to try to get the gum out of my hair. My husband decided that would be a good time to start romancing me by getting into the shower with me.

I informed him that I needed to remove the gum and told him to get out of the shower. The gum tangled painfully in my hair, and my nerves were already frayed from the confrontation at the concert. I got out, wrapped a towel around myself, but he continued to make advances.

I again asked him to stop. I was not in the mood. Dealing with the gum and the entire ordeal had put me in a foul mood. He pushed me down on the bed and held me there against my will.

I screamed, "Stop! Let me up!"

He still persisted.

Fear and anger surged through me at once. I then punched him in the mouth with my closed fist.

This made him mad, so he got up off the bed.

I immediately got up to put my clothes on and told him I was leaving. He threw my tennis shoes and boots across the room to keep me from dressing. The more I insisted on leaving, the angrier he became.

Finally, he said, "You want to play games? I will show you a game."

He put my cell phone in his pocket, and then he called the police with his own phone. I had no phone to call for help, and he was physically blocking the door so I could not leave.

Within ten minutes, the police were there for the call of domestic violence.

My husband was turning the tables on me.

He had to show me who was boss.

The realization of what he was doing hit me with a cold wave of fear. What had just happened inside that room was now being twisted into something else entirely.

The officers questioned us both separately.

The officer who spoke with me was young, his expression professionally neutral. He held a small notepad and wrote as I talked.

"He held me down on the bed," I said. "I told him to stop. I asked him more than once."

The officer wrote something. "Did he strike you?"

"No. He held me. He wouldn't let me up."

"Did you strike him?"

I hesitated. "Yes. I hit him in the mouth. Because he wouldn't let me go."

The officer looked up briefly, then back down at his notepad.

"The gum in my hair, that was from the concert. A woman behind us. And his temple, that was her too. She hit him. I didn't do that." I could hear myself speaking faster, trying to place each injury in its right story. "The marks on his chest are from my boot heels. He had me on his shoulders during the show."

The officer nodded slowly, the way people do when they are listening but have already formed a conclusion.

"He has my phone," I said. "He took it so I couldn't call anyone. Can you ask him for it?"

That, at least, they did. After searching his four pockets, they produced it. Even then, the full meaning of that did not seem to register with them, that a man who lied about the phone might be lying about other things as well.

I stood there and watched the truth leave the room, carried out in the shape of a story that was not mine.

He pointed to the left temple where the woman at the concert had hit him and showed the bruises on his chest from my boots while I had been on his shoulders. Next, he pointed out his lip, where it was swelling from being hit.

He was claiming that all the injuries and bruises were the result of an abusive act by me.

Standing there, I could feel the truth slipping out of my control, my voice small against the carefully arranged story he was presenting.

The cops did not ask me the right questions to get to the truth. If the officers had asked me where I hit him and how, they would have realized he was lying, and my claims of forced sex or rape may have seemed far more reasonable. He denied to the cops that he had my cell phone, but after they searched the four pockets on him, he finally produced it. Even then, the cops still did not see that if he was lying about the phone, he might be lying about other things as well.

I was arrested for DOMESTIC VIOLENCE.

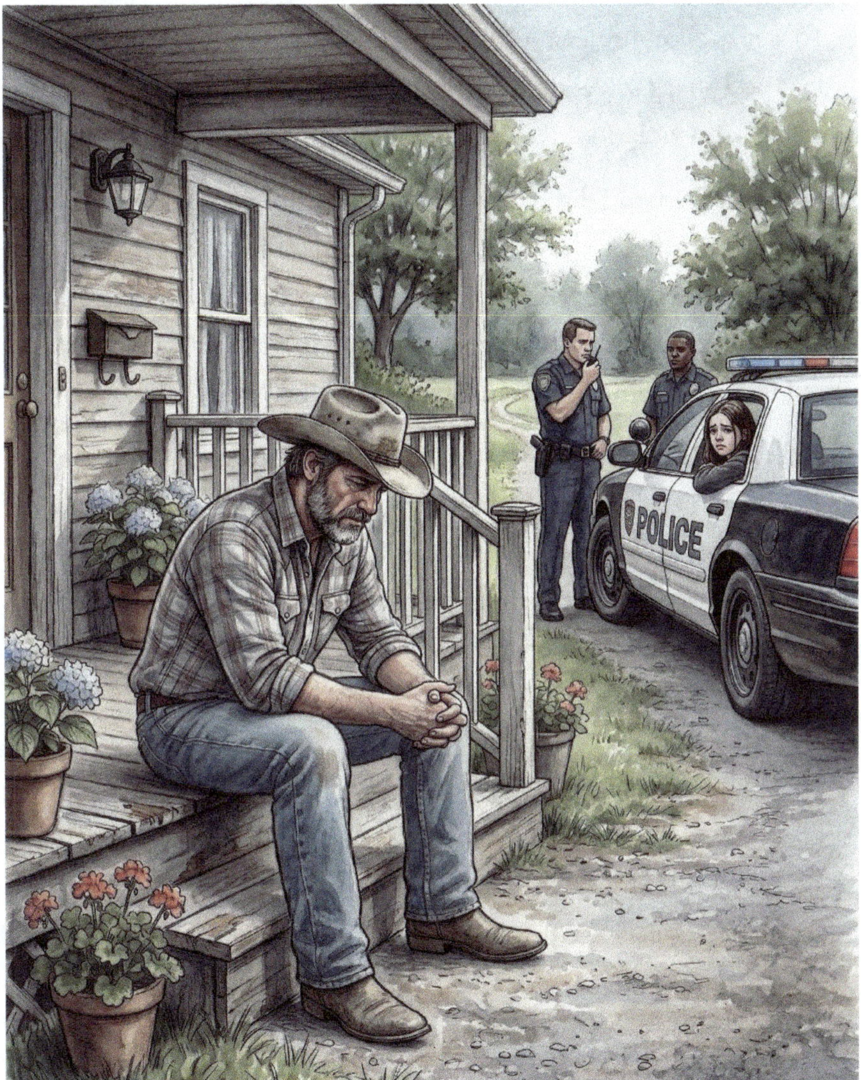

The charge was domestic abuse, and I was taken to the detention center. As they drove off, he sat on the steps of the house and grinned at me, as if the entire situation had become some twisted victory in his mind.

To get a clear understanding of the essence of rape, it must be understood that rape is not just about penetration, and it is not just about physical violation. Rape is a violation of the human spirit.

What my husband did to me, and to all the other women who have since told their stories, showed a complete lack of reverence for another human being, especially for a woman. It revealed his need to feel Godlike, his need for control over others, no matter how much pain it caused us. In his mind, it was just playing a game, no big deal.

Well, it was clearly a big enough deal that my life and the lives of all the other women were changed forever. When he stood up and said, “You want to play games?” and then called the cops, it was a clear message of his character, or rather, his lack of one. What he saw as power and control left lasting damage far beyond that single night.

***

The following evening, I was released. He went to the detention center and paid my bail. He thought that all of this would be just a joke and that he would have shown me “who is in control.”

However, once the bail was paid, the bondsman told him that we could not have contact with each other until the arraignment. The restraining order was for three months. He had actually thought he could simply walk into court, pay the fine, and take me home to continue life as usual.

The bondsman delivered the news with the practiced patience of someone who had said it many times.

"No contact. That means no calls, no texts, no showing up at the residence. Until after the arraignment."

Tom stared at him. "For how long?"

"Three months."

There was a pause. When Tom spoke again, his voice had shifted into the softer register, the one he reached for when he needed something. "She's my wife. I just paid her bail. Surely if she agrees..."

"Sir, it is a court order. Her agreement doesn't change that."

Tom turned and looked at me across the room. I recognized the expression, the calculation beneath the calm, the quick mental inventory of what moves were still available to him. Then his jaw tightened.

He turned back to the bondsman. "Can I at least speak with her before she goes?"

"No."

He could not believe that he would not be able to sweet-talk himself back into my life. He then knew that this might be his final action as a husband. He begged the constable to let me go home with him so we could talk. He was again informed that there would be no talking until after the arraignment. He was losing the battle, but he would not let that happen without trying to regain control.

I went to the orphanage for safety. For the first time in a long while, those familiar walls felt like refuge rather than memory. Chase had come home on leave and had Chason with him, so at least my little boy was safe with his father. Though exhausted, humiliated, and emotionally shaken, I felt a small sense of relief knowing that for the moment, Chason and I were out of immediate danger.

Becky opened the door before I had finished knocking. She took one look at me and stepped aside without a word.

I walked in and stood in the hallway, not sure my legs would carry me any further. The smell of the place, the wood and the warmth and the faint trace of something always baking, pressed against me like a hand on my back.

"I didn't know where else to go," I said.

"You came home," Becky said simply.

She put both arms around me, the way she had done since I was small enough to fit in a crib, and held on. I did not cry right away. I stood very still for a moment, the way a person does when they have been holding themselves together for so long that they have forgotten what it feels like not to.

Then I did cry. And Becky held on.

She did not ask me anything that night. She brought me tea and a blanket and sat with me until I was quiet. There would be time for questions later. For now, it was enough that I was here.

Tom was not satisfied with giving up on me, even though it could be temporary. He was mad. He went back to our home and proceeded to remove all of my clothing, my pictures, the video camera, the baby seat, the video player, my debit card, my money, my ID, the wedding certificate, and other legal documents. The removal was not random.

It was deliberate, methodical, and intended to leave me with nothing. He even went to the jewelry repair shop where my wedding rings were being sized and picked them up to keep.

He called his brother to come and get the Hummer. He then allowed them to vacation across the East Coast in my car. I was left without a vehicle to transport myself and Chason for three weeks. To him, this was punishment. In his mind, he was "teaching me a lesson." Revenge was sweet to him.

The following day, my lawyer filed a petition with the court for him to return all personal belongings belonging to me and Chason.

His explanation to the court was, "They must have gotten mixed in with his clothes."

The excuse was almost absurd. The video camera? The DVD player? The pictures? The car seat? Yet he continued to spin his tale, continuing his lies with the same confidence that had carried him this far. It was unsettling how easily he could still convince others.

I was planning on attending my friend's graduation. He returned the rings so I could wear them in public and show that I was married. Even then, he was still under the impression that he could say anything, lie about everything, and get by with it. After six months of this drama, however, his lies were becoming easier for most people to recognize.

This little stunt of his cost him $5,000.00 for his lawyer. My attorney cost $3,750.00.

I used my rings as collateral.

The symbolism of that did not escape me. The very rings that had once represented promises and hope were now being used simply to survive and protect myself.

I got my own cell phone so that he could no longer track me. However, after turning my old phone off and later back on again, he realized that the phone had been his only contact with me. He started texting me and calling me on the old phone, but I did not respond.

His attorney informed him that within thirty days, he must return the vehicle to me and pay for my living expenses.

He returned the Hummer in the fourth week and put $1,000.00 in a bank account for me, upon instructions from his attorney. After three weeks of no money, no transportation, and no food other than what was given to me by others, he avoided being put in jail for failing to take care of me by complying within the month's time limit.

My next step was to file criminal charges against him for neglect.

His attorney had informed him of this possibility, but it had not yet been thirty days. I would have to wait until the full thirty days had passed, and then I could file charges.

Finally, it began to register with Cowboy Tom that he had to act like a responsible husband, or at the very least, a responsible person.

It was four weeks by the fifth of July.

He went to the house, cut the lawn, wrote a check for the rent, and paid the utilities. He put one hundred dollars on the debit card for me to live on.

Even these actions felt less like care and more like obligation, done only because legal consequences were beginning to close in around him.

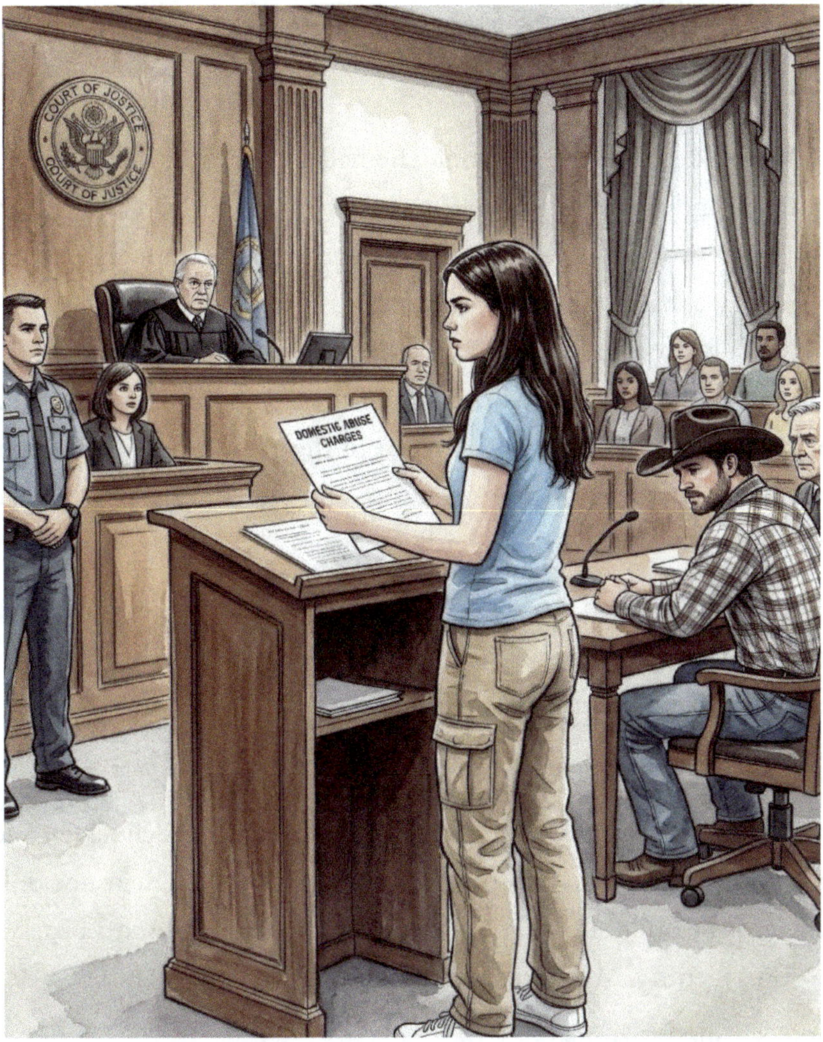

It was now arraignment day.

I pleaded not guilty, and a court date was set.

The weight of that moment settled heavily on me. Unless this charge was removed from my record, it would always remain there, a permanent mark tied to a lie that had already taken so much from me.

CHAPTER FOUR

When I returned to my home, he had moved out. I checked the contents, and everything seemed to be returned that had been taken. For a brief moment, I felt a small measure of relief, thinking perhaps the damage had only been temporary. Then, when I went into Chason's bedroom, I looked at the heritage quilt I had hung on the wall, the one that displayed pictures of my friends and animals from the orphanage. It had always been one of the most treasured things in the room, filled with memory, comfort, and pieces of the life that had shaped me.

One picture stood out as not fitting in the way the others did. Then I realized that someone had taken a Q-tip dipped in bleach and whited out the face of Chason's father in the picture.

I broke down in tears.

Only one person would do something so cruel, so deliberate, and so unkind. The act felt deeply personal, as though he had not only damaged the quilt but had tried to erase a part of my life and a part of my son's identity. My heart was broken.

The quilt was ruined.

What would I tell my friends?

Penny came over that afternoon and found me sitting on the edge of Chason's bed, the quilt folded in my lap, my hands resting still on top of it. She did not need to ask what had happened. She could see.

"Oh, Tera," she said quietly, sitting down beside me.

I did not look up. “It was the bleach. He used a Q-tip.”

Penny was silent for a moment. Then she said, very carefully, “That was not an accident.”

“I know.”

“That was done on purpose, to hurt you.”

“I know that too.” I smoothed my hand across the faded square where Chase’s face used to be. “Becky made this for me. The girls all sewed it together.” My voice broke on the last word.

Penny put her arm around me and held on. She did not say anything else. There was nothing left to say that the ruined quilt had not already said far more plainly.

***

MANIPULATION

Once I was home, the telephone calls started up again. Always, with a loving, kind voice, he would beg to come home. His tone was soft, apologetic, and filled with the kind of warmth that once had made me feel safe. I was lonesome. The quiet of the house, though peaceful at times, also left space for loneliness to creep in. He was persuasive. He vowed never to do anything to hurt me again.

The whirlwind romance started up again.

What had once felt like destiny was actually a carefully orchestrated psychological campaign designed to make me feel emotionally dependent on him. The fairy-tale beginning had become the setup for a nightmare, yet in moments of loneliness, it was hard for me to see that clearly.

The calls always came in the evening, after Chason was in bed and the house had gone quiet. That was when loneliness pressed hardest.

His voice, when he called, was always the gentle one. The one I had fallen for.

"I miss you," he said. "I miss hearing you in the house. I miss the way you laugh."

I did not answer right away. I was pressing the phone against my ear and staring at the wall.

"You hurt me," I said at last.

"I know I did. And I will spend the rest of my life making it up to you if you let me. I've changed, Tera. I know you probably don't believe that. But I have."

There was something in the quiet after those words that I could not fill fast enough. "How do I know?"

"Because I'm asking," he said. "A man who doesn't care doesn't ask. He just disappears. I'm still here. I'm still calling."

I pressed my fingers against my eyes. The argument made a kind of sense that I could feel even as some quieter part of me knew it should not. That was the part I could not listen to yet.

I was enjoying being home with just Chason. He was starting to talk in full sentences, keeping me laughing at his little words and the sweet way he said them. Those small moments with him brought genuine joy back into my days. Friends were visiting me once again, and I loved it. They always seemed to have a little gift with them for Chason. I felt lucky, almost as though life was trying to give me a second chance at happiness.

Finally, his persuasions paid off.

He had discovered exactly where my weakness lay and continued with more lies and promises. It only took two months.

After two months, Bubba Tom begged to move back in with me. I was missing him, and in my loneliness, the memories of his abuse had begun to fade behind the memory of his warm touch and his carefully chosen words.

I wanted to see his ranch.

I wanted to see the horses.

So, I agreed.

Lately, he had only kind, loving words toward me. He made it sound like the past had not happened, that it was mostly my imagination that caused the problems.

He soon moved back into the house with the promise of moving me to the ranch. Two months later, he finally started packing our belongings into the horse trailer and said we were moving to the ranch.

Except there was no ranch.

I was so excited with anticipation. Finally, we would have our own home, and I could ride the horses I had dreamed about for so long.

I kept looking at the scenery as we drove. With excitement building inside me, I could hardly wait.

Tom pulled into a driveway off the highway in front of a shotgun-style house that badly needed paint. It had a tree in front and a couple of hedges beneath the window.

This must be the barn, I thought.

Where is the house?

I kept peeking around, still searching for the ranch house he had promised me, expecting at any moment to see open fields, fencing, horses, and the life he had painted so vividly in his words.

He stopped the truck.

In that moment, the weight of realization began to settle over me.

He knew I had a deep well of longing inside me that had never truly been filled, a longing for home, for permanence, for belonging, for the dream I had carried since childhood.

And he had used it.

I would accept this, he believed.

He immediately started making warm remarks, knowing I would listen.

"This is your new home," he said. "I will make this into the home you always wanted. When I finish remodeling, you will love it."

I was shocked.

He had spotted the invisible wound that made me crave the very thing I had never received as a child. He could see the way I lit up when someone paid attention to me, how grateful I became for even basic kindness, and how quickly I forgave behavior that should have sent anyone running. He had a way of explaining things that made me believe he was sincere. The blood drained from my face as the reality of what stood before me began to settle in.

I got out of the truck, still puzzled that this was what he was calling a ranch. My head was swimming with disbelief, not knowing what to say or do. I kept looking around, almost expecting that perhaps the real house was hidden somewhere beyond the trees or behind the structure in front of me.

I stood at the truck door, not yet able to make myself move toward it. The words were out of my mouth before I had time to soften them.

"Tom. This is a barn."

He continued with his story.

“It’s a house,” he said patiently, as though I were the one misunderstanding. “It just needs some work. You know I can do the work.”

“You told me a ranch. You said horses. You said...”

“And we will have all of that.” He came around the side of the truck and stood beside me, his voice dropping into the gentle register I had come to depend on. “This is where it starts, Tera. Not where it ends. Can you trust me on that?”

I looked at the structure in front of me. The peeling paint. The flat, featureless face of it. Then I looked at him.

And I wanted to believe him so badly that I let myself.

“Okay,” I said. The word came out barely above a whisper.

He smiled and put his arm around my shoulders, and we walked toward the barn door together as though it were a front porch.

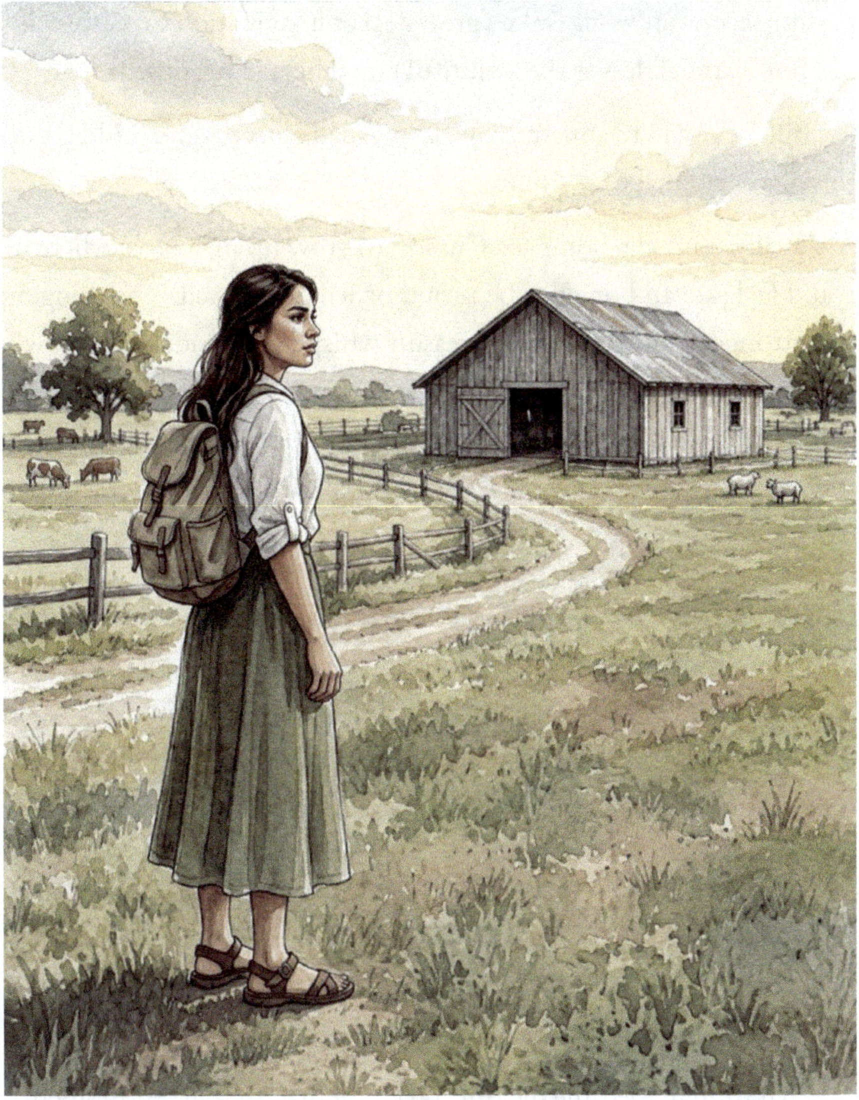

I had moved from my home, believing I was moving to a better place. I soon found out that this shack was on property owned by his parents, and it could never be mistaken for a ranch-style home. It was a hay barn. He had moved his bed and a table into it and had been living there when he met me. The truth struck me harder with every passing second. It would take a great deal of imagination to picture this as a home, much less as the beautiful ranch he had promised.

Still, he began to convince me, to persuade me, that he could fix up this place and make it a home.

I really wanted a home for Chason to grow up in, a place where he could feel safe and one day be proud of where he lived. That longing was stronger than the voice of reason whispering inside me. I slowly and quietly accepted the situation, still believing this was temporary, still waiting for the butterflies to continue to flutter in my stomach, as if hope itself could somehow transform the truth.

I became pregnant.

I should have been happy, but the drama I had been living in had cast a fog over my joy. Instead of excitement, what I felt most was uncertainty. The thought of bringing another child into such instability weighed heavily on my heart. I started praying silently and quietly, hoping with everything inside me that life would somehow become better.

I settled into a routine, almost as if I had given up, yet I was still holding on to hope.

Maybe when this baby is born, things will be better, I imagined.

That thought became the thread I clung to in the darkest moments, the small promise I repeated to myself when reality became too painful to face.

I was still holding out for hope.

"I have faith," I would say out loud.

Although there was no one there to hear me, speaking the words aloud made them feel more real, as though saying them could keep me from falling apart.

I was too embarrassed to call Becky.

Becky was the one person who would have understood, the one person who would have seen through the promises and the lies. But I kept my secret life a secret from all the people who mattered most to me. My feelings of confusion and distress caused me to feel guilty and ashamed.

I told no one.

A month or two later, he did some things to the house to make it livable, such as turning the oversized room he had been using as a bedroom into two smaller ones. It was not much, but to me, any change that hinted at permanence felt like progress. The kitchen floors still had only plywood for flooring, as did the bathroom. Sheets were hung on the windows, with no blinds or drapes to soften the harshness of the place. The house still carried the feel of something unfinished, something temporary, despite all the promises that had been made.

Later, my friends from the home bought blinds for the living room to replace the sheets. Their kindness touched me, but their concern was evident. They could not understand why I remained with him. To them, it was a very disturbing sight, not only because of the condition of the house but also because they did not know how to help me fix things or make it better. They could see the cracks in the life I was trying so hard to believe in. Still, I continued believing in him, regardless of the lies. He had promised me a home, a ranch with horses, and I held tightly to that vision.

Still living within his lies, he again promised me a new home. He contacted a draftsman and had a lovely home designed, complete with blueprints. He gave me the blueprints and had me start contacting contractors to build the home. Holding those plans in my hands felt like finally touching the future I had dreamed of. He began grading land for the house to be built on and worked several days shaping it into a pad for the house.

I was so excited. I ran to him and hugged him tightly. "Thank you, thank you," I proclaimed. "You make me so happy."

He grinned. But nothing was said. That silence should have meant something, yet I chose to fill it with hope.

I called Becky and told her of the plans. Becky held her breath, remembering the way he had treated me in the past, and became afraid for me. Even through the joy in my voice, Becky could hear the same fragile hope that had been broken before.

What I did not know was that he was grading land on his parents' property. He knew he was not building a home there. It was part of his game, another carefully crafted deception that I turned a blind eye toward. It was not his property. It was another lie. No one in his family told me of the deception.

They all knew. Still, I held on to hope. Soon it was nearly time for the baby to be born. I called Becky.

"I think I need to go to the hospital. I am cramping, but the pains are not real close yet. Can you come get me?"

Becky was so excited that I had called her. The call meant trust, and perhaps, in Becky's heart, a chance to be there for me again in the way she had always longed to be. She hurriedly dressed and was on her way.

When Becky arrived, she was surprised to see Tom's mother's car in the driveway.

I came to the door and announced, "Sheila is here, so she can drive me. I am sorry I bothered you. I will call you later and let you know when the baby is born."

Becky was puzzled. She said, "It is no bother. I was looking forward to being with you."

There was hurt beneath her words, though she tried to hide it. Sheila came outside and said, "I am here now. I will take care of her. You can go home, and we will call you later."

Becky left, trying to stop the tears. As she drove away, the ache in her heart deepened, not only from being turned away but from the growing feeling that I was slipping further into a life no one could reach.

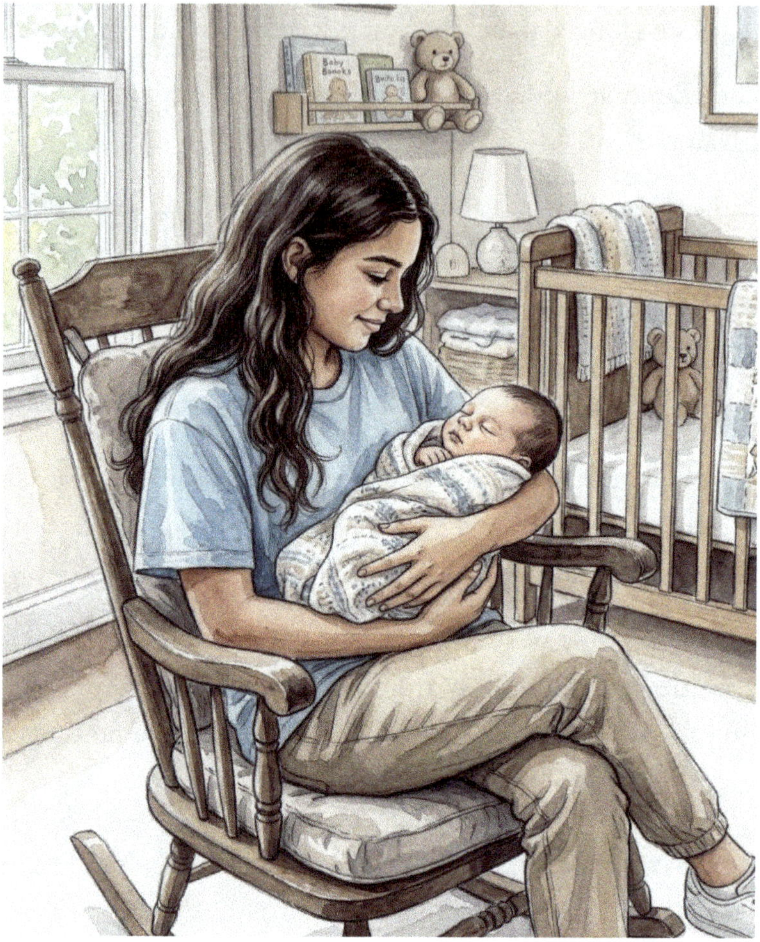

Soon, I was home with the new baby boy, named Tyler, but Becky did not receive an invitation to come see the baby or to visit. She simply got a phone call telling her that the baby had been born, was healthy, and that I was okay. The call was brief, carrying the news but none of the warmth Becky had once shared with me. For Becky, it was another painful reminder of the distance that had grown between us.

Two months went by, and Tom said that the contractors would be calling for an appointment to start the project.

I was so excited that he was getting the land ready for the contractors to begin laying the foundation. In my mind, this was the moment everything would finally begin to come together. I could almost picture the walls rising, the rooms taking shape, and a real home forming around my children. But no one came.

I waited.

When I questioned Tom about the delay, he answered, "It is a busy season. We are on his list to start, but we have to wait our turn."

So, I continued to wait, my anxious feelings mixed with excitement. Each day I listened for the sound of trucks, for footsteps at the door, for any sign that the dream was beginning.

Six more months went by, and construction had still not begun.

He gave me the answer that the plans needed to be revised and that it would take time, but the original plans were still lying on the table in the hall, untouched except for the dust that had begun to settle over them.

Instead, he went back to the draftsman and had him draw another set of plans, this time remodeling the hay-shed house by adding more rooms and moving walls to accommodate a family's home. This was not discussed with me. I was still believing I was getting a real home for my growing family, but it was just another farce, unknown to me.

I looked at the plans and tried to be happy with the new arrangement of the hay house, still not sure of what to believe.

I thought, *maybe it will make a nice home. I have to have faith.* I wanted to believe.

He had no intentions of building a home on his parents' property, where he had spent weekends grading the property. It was still all part of his long psychological game. Every new plan, every revised drawing, every small change was enough to keep hope alive inside me. But I still had a blind heart to his game. I did not question him about all the changes. Whenever doubt tried to surface, he would pour just enough love and attention over me to fill that lonely feeling buried so deep inside.

My friends began to talk to me about the situation. They could see what I was unable or unwilling to see.

He, too, was talking to me about my friends.

Slowly, he began to isolate me from them, turning partial truths into total lies. He twisted their concern into criticism and their love into interference. I was listening to him and listening less to my friends.

Tom said, "We have to get on another list with another contractor. The last one moved to another state and did not leave the plans and list of clients behind." (I later found out that it was not true.)

Again, there was another reason to wait.

During the next six months, as I waited, he began to remodel the existing bathroom by putting in a sink and a built-in cabinet. He was doing just enough work on the hay house to keep me believing in him. Each small improvement felt like proof to me that maybe this time, things were moving forward.

It took a few months working on it, and I was satisfied that he was working toward the remodeled home plan.

I had not yet seen the pattern of his games. Every delay came with an excuse. Every excuse came with just enough action. And every small action kept hope alive.

Six more months went by, and he built a full-length porch on the back of the hay-house. All this time, the house was not even his to be building onto; it belonged to his parents. There was no one else who would have fallen for what he was doing, but I did. With each lie, he was also convincing me that I should stay away from my orphanage friends.

I was no longer consulting with friends and family who might have pointed out the concerning behaviors. My early relationship with Tom had become the most dangerous part of love because it had rewritten my understanding of what love should feel like. He had showered me with more affection in two months than I had received in my entire teen life. He was taking advantage of the trauma bond that had formed, an emotional addiction to the highs and lows of the relationship. When he showed up offering what seemed like unlimited love and acceptance, my heart and mind interpreted it as the very thing I had been waiting for my entire life. The intensity did not feel unhealthy to me, because intensity had become the only way I knew how to recognize love.

Chason continued to tell me how Tom was treating him when I was not looking or when I was not around. Each time, my little boy's voice carried confusion and hurt, hoping I would finally hear him. When Tom came in from work, he spotted Chason and seemed to interpret the child's very presence as an interference to the family life he wanted to control. His face turned red with anger.

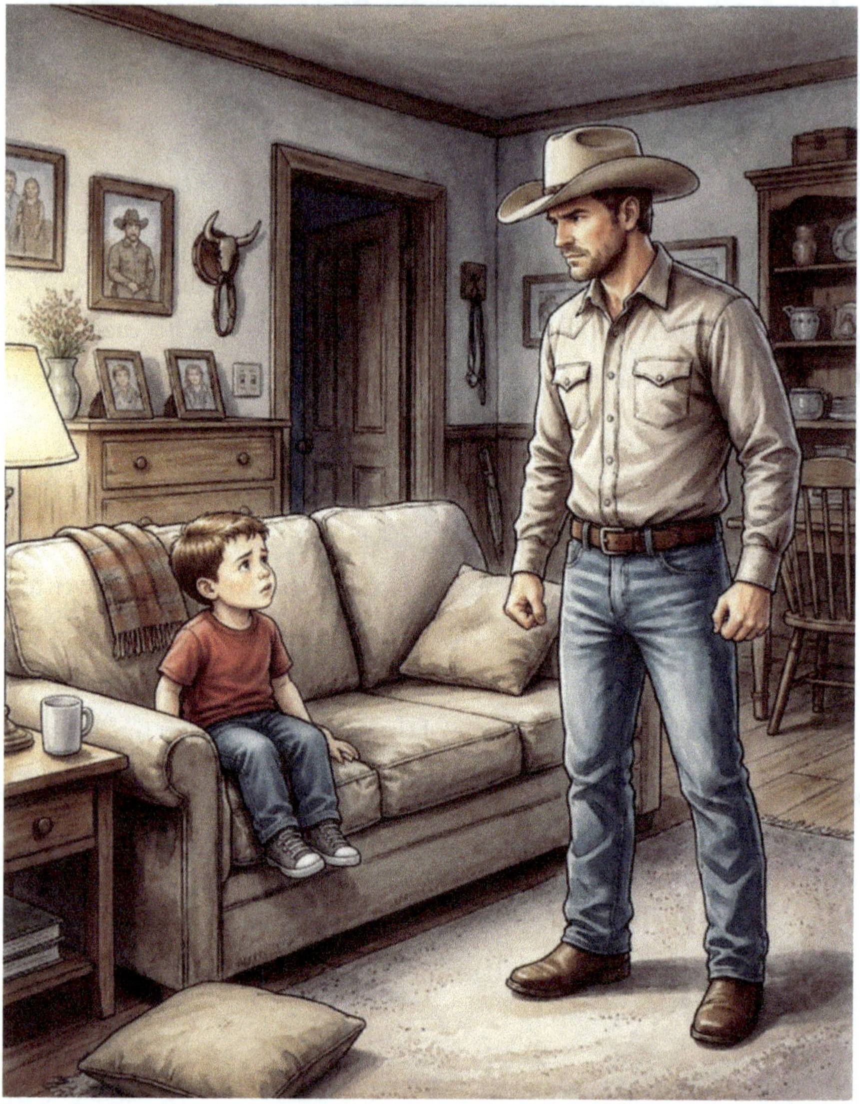

He picked up Chason and threw him onto the sofa, causing him to bounce off and fall to the floor. Penny was there, sitting in the dining room where Tom could not see her. She saw everything. Chason ran to me crying, his small face wet with tears, but Tom was right behind him, quickly telling the version of events he wanted me to believe. Penny knew at once that he was lying, that he had physically abused Chason by throwing him. But he was believable, or at least I desperately wanted to believe him. To Penny's disbelief, I even laughed softly, brushing aside the incident as if it were nothing. I did not truly look at my son's distressed face. I only saw Tom.

Later, when Tom had gone outside and Chason was watching television in the next room, Penny found me at the kitchen sink. She kept her voice low but did not soften it.

"Tera, I need you to hear me."

"Penny, it was nothing. He just..."

"I was sitting right there." Her voice did not rise, but it was steady as stone. "I saw what he did. He picked that boy up and threw him. That is not playing. That is not rough-housing. That is a grown man throwing a child."

I kept my eyes on the water running over my hands. "Chase overreacts sometimes. You know how boys..."

"Don't." The word came out quietly but it stopped me cold. Penny set her hand on my arm. "I know what I saw. And part of you knows it too. I can see it in your face right now."

I turned the tap off. My hands were trembling slightly, though I hoped she could not tell.

"It won't happen again," I said.

Penny looked at me for a long moment. There was no anger in her eyes. Only something much sadder. "It already did," she said gently. "That's what 'again' means."

She left shortly after. I stood at the sink a long time after she was gone, staring at nothing, filling the silence with reasons instead of truth.

The new baby boy seemed to escape his tantrums. He appeared to enjoy the new child, holding him and speaking gently in ways that made me believe there was goodness still in him. That, too, became another excuse not to pay attention to Chason and the pain he was quietly carrying.

After a while, Chason stopped telling me what was happening. When Penny or Becky questioned him as to why he had stopped telling me, he answered in a small, defeated voice, "She doesn't believe me. She believes him."

Becky had been the one who finally drew it out of him. She had found him sitting alone on the back step of the orphanage during a visit, apart from the other children, his eyes fixed on something that was not there.

"Hey, you," she said softly, settling down beside him the way she had once sat beside me.

Chason did not answer right away.

"You can tell me," Becky said. "You always could."

He picked at a loose thread on the hem of his shirt. "She doesn't believe me," he said at last, barely above a whisper. "She believes him."

Becky did not rush to fill the silence. She let the words sit for a moment, let them be heard.

"I believe you," she said finally. "I want you to know that. Whatever you have told me, whatever you haven't, I believe you."

He looked up at her then. His eyes were steady in the way that broke her heart, the kind of steady that does not come from strength but from having already learned there was no point in falling apart.

Then he looked away again, and neither of them said anything more.

Penny and Becky were heartbroken for my little boy. No child should have been forced to live with that sort of treatment, nor with the crushing realization that the person meant to protect him would not listen. Their hearts ached for him, knowing he was learning far too early what it meant to feel unseen and unheard in his own home.

Becky contacted Chase's mother and confided in her about what had happened. Becky asked his mother if she was going to tell Chase. She replied, "Oh no, Chase would kill him!" So Chason's father was not aware of what was going on. Chason only confided in Becky and Penny. They knew the truth, and the burden of carrying that truth weighed heavily on both of them.

It was now three and a half years later. Six more months had gone by. He bought five acres of land from his parents, located in front of their house, about three hundred feet away. He told me he needed the acreage for his horses to roam. In reality, he was preparing me for the letdown that he knew would come when he finally told me of his plans.

"We can go shopping for a triple-wide mobile home and move it onto the property, with the horses on the land with us," I excitedly stated. My eyes brightened at the thought, and for the first time in a long while, hope stirred in my heart again.

He let me think that we could purchase a triple-wide manufactured home and place it on the five acres. I was once again filled with excitement, believing that we were finally going to move out of the hay-house and into a beautiful home. We went to the nearest large town, looking at homes, and finally, after several shopping trips, I found the one I wanted. I could already picture the rooms, where the children would sleep, where the kitchen table would sit, and where I might finally feel proud to welcome people inside.

We went to the bank.

He now had to find a way to avoid buying the triple-wide. While speaking with the banker, he suddenly decided that a mortgage was not what he wanted, and he refused to buy the home. He refused the financing, telling me he was saving toward a home and that it would not be long before he could pay cash for it. The words fell heavily on my heart. I left crying, the excitement of the day collapsing into yet another deep disappointment.

We met Becky for dinner on the way back to our home. I was still upset, trying to hold back tears, and I told Becky that he would not get the home for me after all.

Becky set her fork down and looked at me across the table. She chose her words the way she always did, slowly and without sharpness, though I could see the effort it cost her.

"Tera," she said quietly. "How many times now has the home been promised?"

I looked at my plate. "He said he'll save for it. Pay cash. He says a mortgage isn't..."

"That isn't what I asked." Her voice was gentle, but it did not move. "I asked how many times it's been promised."

I did not answer. I reached for my glass instead.

Becky watched me for a moment. She did not press. She had learned a long time ago that pressing too hard only pushed me further from reach. But before we left the table that evening, she laid her hand over mine and held it for a moment.

"I am always here," she said. "When you're ready. I am always here."

He had played me one more time. Even then, I soon accepted his lies and accepted my situation. I really wanted to believe. I really wanted to make the marriage work. More than anything, I wanted to believe that the life I had dreamed of was still possible.

Christmas came, and I was still in the hay-house. I was devastated that things were not what I had thought they would be. The disappointment had begun to settle into something heavier, something harder to ignore. We were arguing and fighting over these issues more often now. He knew I was almost giving up and might leave him.

So, he promised me that when the child support to his oldest daughter was over, he would get me a home. That would be in less than five years.

Would I wait that long?

Maybe it was the darkness closing in around me, or maybe it was finally the light I was beginning to see.

I left for a week to visit friends in Texas. When I returned, there was a single-wide used trailer sitting on the acreage in front of his parents' home. He had moved the trailer onto the property and said, "Here is your home!"

The words struck me in silence. I stood there staring at it, not knowing whether to cry, scream, or simply go numb. This was not the dream he had painted for me. This was not the home he had promised. Yet once again, he had presented disappointment as if it were a gift.

I was shocked.

He was once again the man in control, and I would live the way he wanted, and I did. *What? This is my home? No triple-wide? A 12x45 used trailer?* The disbelief settled over me like a cold weight. The dream he had built in my mind had once again been reduced to something far smaller, far sadder, than what he had promised.

I now had a single-wide, out in the woods, in front of his parents' home. He was a happy camper. I was not. He could go off to work, knowing his parents could keep an eye on me. Since he cheated and lied, surely in his mind, I must be doing the same. He had now separated me from my friends, the only family I had ever truly known. The love and support they could provide to me and my children was now almost lost.

He had skillfully managed to influence me in a deceptive, selfish, and unfair manner. I had not yet seen it for what it was. The lingering effects from the petit-mal diagnosis kept me feeling like a prisoner, uncertain of what to do or even what to think. The damage may have been minor, but it was enough that he took advantage of the situation, using my confusion and vulnerability to keep me under his control.

Almost overnight, the visiting with my friends, and their visits with me, had stopped. The silence around my life had grown louder than any words. Chason was getting older now, and like me, he too was beginning to adjust to the mental abuse as if it were normal. There was no one for him to tell his fears to. No one was coming around anymore. He still had his dad, but the fear that his Mimi had instilled in him of what his dad would do if he ever knew the truth kept him silent.

He could not tell me about Papa Tom pinning him to the floor. Chason and Tyler had been wrestling on the floor, laughing and having fun like little boys should, but Papa Tom decided that Chason was being too rough with his son and chose to intervene in cruelty rather than care. He pinned him down on the floor, hands around his neck, and said the chilling words, "I will make you wish you were never born!"

Tyler later repeated this to Becky while visiting the school for Family Day. All Becky could do was wrap her arms around the boys' necks and hold them close, tears filling her eyes as she realized the abuse they were enduring behind closed doors. Chason looked up at Becky with eyes far too old for a child and said, "I don't think Papa loves me."

Becky looked at him and knew his little heart was broken. The sadness in his voice, the quiet acceptance in his face, told her more than words ever could. No child should ever have to question whether he is loved.

Finally, Tom started laying his final plans. We were now living in the small trailer instead of the roomy hay-house. Tom began to think that I might be waking up to his deceptions. So, he said to me, "Let's move the hay-house over here and remodel it just the way you want, or like it to be."

He continued to enhance the likelihood that I would love the new home when it was finished. Three more years went by, and we were still in the small trailer, but I was adapting to my position. I was doing everything I could to keep the peace, with that inner desire for love still longing for my heart to be filled. I had the two boys and loved every minute with them, yet I had begun to grow restless. A quiet emptiness had started to settle inside me. I felt that something was missing, but I was not sure what it was. Maybe a job outside of the house would help. Maybe being around other people again would remind me of who I used to be.

Years passed, and Chason was now twelve. He joined the football team. The first two years that a student was with the team were basically for learning, observing, exercising, and doing all the rituals of the team. The first time to actually walk onto the field and play would occur in the third year. He was waiting for his turn, holding onto that moment with quiet determination.

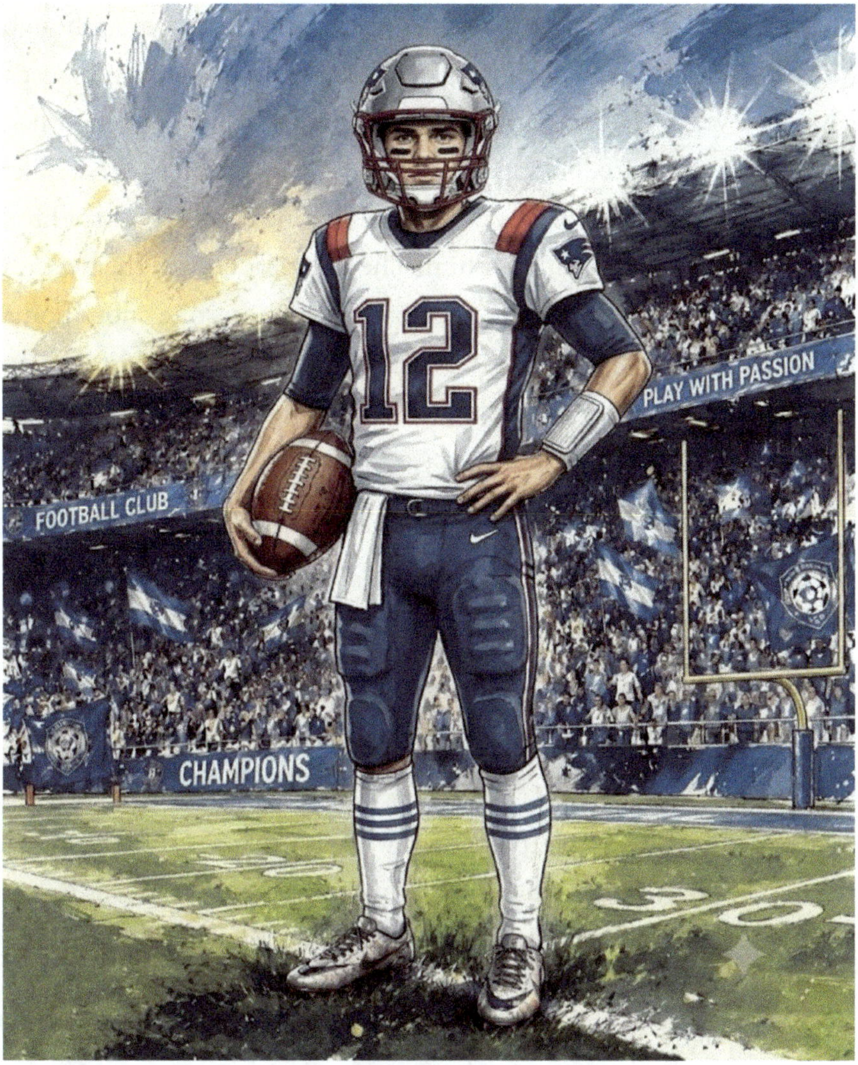

Pictures of Chason appeared on the school roster, wearing his number proudly. He could hardly wait another two years, so he could finally play. He was learning patience along with the plays and practices. Each practice, each drill, and each game he watched from the bench became part of his preparation, and he carried himself with a maturity that made everyone notice him.

My friends would go to the games just to see Chason, even though he was sitting on the bench each game. They understood that in just a couple of years, they would finally get to see him play. Chason had developed into a nice-looking young man, tall and strong, with a quiet presence that drew people toward him. Everyone was so proud of him. Everyone was there rooting for him. The cheerleaders had their eye on him as well. Everyone wanted to get to know him. In spite of our home life, he had grown into a fine person. He was basically limited to church activities and very few school functions, yet somehow, he continued to carry himself with grace and restraint.

Chason asked for a cell phone. He was told, "No, not until you are sixteen!"

He had friends who let him use their phones whenever he needed a ride home from practice. He had learned to be patient, telling himself that someday things would be better. Someday, he would be old enough to make his own choices.

It became quite noticeable to all my friends that the two boys were treated differently. But Chason's outward appearance did not reflect disappointment. He had learned how to hide his hurt behind silence. Inside, however, he would quietly plead with himself that one day he would be eighteen. That seemed to be a magic number to him, a doorway to freedom, a future where he might finally be able to breathe without fear.

I look back at this now and wonder how could I have been so blind?

When his younger brother, Tyler, wanted a phone, he was given one at age thirteen. Chason was also given one at the same time, but only because they had waited until he was sixteen, or rather, waited until

Tyler had asked for one. Then suddenly it was acceptable. I went along with Tom's direction.

The difference in how they were treated did not go unnoticed by Chason. He said little, but each moment settled quietly into his heart, another reminder of where he stood in the household. Why did I not notice?

Tyler had the same love for horses as I did. Chason had no desire to have a horse, nor to ride one, nor to live on a ranch. Inwardly, he was already shaping his own future, and it did not include his past. He was told by both me and his stepfather, "You are not trying to fit in!" Yet no one ever asked, "What do you want with your life?" So, he kept silent and attended his church functions, hoping to find some understanding of his life there, some peace that he could not seem to find at home.

I seemed to find comfort in the church and in the friendships of the church ladies. Slowly, my old friends were becoming part of my past. The distance between who I had once been and who I had become was growing wider, though I hardly noticed it myself.

I applied for a job as an assistant to the teachers at the boys' school. That became my escape from what had come to feel like a life of captivity. I was still isolated, living in a trailer in front of my in-laws' home. There was very little I could do to escape their constant awareness and quiet monitoring of my activities. I would tend the horses, but seldom got to ride them. That seemed to be what Tom did best, keeping the appearance of giving me what I loved while still withholding the freedom to truly enjoy it.

I began work at the school, loving every moment of it. The children were a delight. Stepping into that classroom each morning felt like stepping into air I could actually breathe.

On the fifth day, trouble found me.

Chason had been complaining of a sore throat all week. I had been treating him with the medicine the doctor had prescribed over the phone, watching him carefully each morning before sending him to school, hoping each day would be better than the last. By Friday, it was clear that it was not.

He was pale and glassy-eyed at breakfast, and when I pressed the back of my hand to his forehead, the heat that met my fingers told me everything I needed to know.

"My throat hurts, Mama," he said, in that small, hoarse voice children use when they are trying not to complain but cannot help it.

"I know, baby. I know." I kissed the top of his head and sat down at the table beside him, thinking.

Five days into a new job. I could not ask for time off. Not yet. Not this soon. I needed this job too much, in too many ways.

There was only one person I trusted without question.

I called Becky.

"Becky, I'm sorry to ask this. I know it's early."

"Tera, stop apologizing and tell me what you need." Her voice was already awake, already steady. She had always been like that.

"Chason is sick. I think it's more than a cold. I've called ahead to the doctor and they're expecting him, but I can't take him myself. I just started at the school and I—"

"I'm on my way," Becky said simply.

"Becky..."

"I'll be there within the hour. You go to work. I'll take care of him."

She arrived exactly when she said she would. She came inside, looked at Chason with the practiced eye of a woman who had assessed sick children for decades, and gently helped him into his jacket. He went with her willingly, leaning slightly against her arm.

"You're going to be just fine," Becky told him, adjusting his collar. "We'll get you to the doctor, and then you can rest. I make very good soup, if I do say so myself."

Chason managed a small smile. "With crackers?"

"With as many crackers as you want."

I stood at the door and watched them walk to her car. There was a tightness in my chest, the working mother's particular guilt of needing to be in two places and being unable to split yourself in half. But underneath it was something steadier. Gratitude. The deep, uncomplicated kind.

"Thank you," I called after her.

Becky looked back and waved her hand as if to say, *Don't be silly,* and got in the car.

I went to work. And I knew he was safe.

***

Becky called me on my lunch break.

"Strep throat," she said. "The doctor gave him a shot and a prescription. He'll need to be kept home for three days."

"Three days," I repeated. My stomach dropped.

"Tera, listen to me. I can keep him. He can stay with me through the weekend, and I will bring him back to you on Monday after school. By then, the amoxicillin should have him feeling like himself again. You do not need to worry."

I closed my eyes for a moment. "Becky, you've already done so much."

"Stop," she said firmly, in that tone she had used since I was small, the one that meant the conversation was settled. "He is my child too. Now go back to your classroom. He is in good hands."

I knew she was right. I had always been able to count on Becky. That was as true on this Friday afternoon as it had been on every day of my life before it.

***

What happened between Friday and Monday, I cannot fully explain, except to say that Tom was home that weekend, and Tom was never idle when there was a thought he wanted to plant.

It started quietly, the way it always did.

Saturday evening, sitting at the table, he said it almost offhandedly, as if it were a passing thought rather than something he had been building toward.

"You know, it's a little strange," he said. "The way Becky inserts herself into things."

I looked up. “She is helping us. She is helping me.”

“I know, I know.” He held up a hand, the picture of reasonableness. “I’m just saying… a woman who has never had her own children, who raises other people’s children her whole life…you have to wonder what that does to a person. What she gets out of it.”

I said nothing.

“She’s very attached to Chason,” he continued. “Always has been. Don’t you think that’s a little too much? He’s your son, Tera. Not hers.”

“She loves him,” I said. “That’s all that is.”

“I’m sure she does.” He picked up his fork again, nodding slowly. “I just want you to be careful. People who love other people’s children that much sometimes start to believe they have a right to them. That’s all I’m saying.”

He did not say anything more about it that night.

He did not need to.

The next morning, Sunday, he came into the kitchen while I was making coffee and said, almost as if he had been worrying about it overnight, “You don’t think she’d try to push for some kind of custody arrangement, do you? I’ve heard of that happening. A grandparent figure, spending enough time with a child, builds a case. You might want to look into that.”

I turned from the counter. “Becky would never…”

“Of course, not intentionally,” he said gently. “But intentions and actions are not always the same thing. I just think you should be careful. That's all. I love you. I'm looking out for you."

In my heart, I knew better.

In my heart, I knew exactly who Becky was, and exactly what she had given Chason and me without ever once asking for anything in return.

But Tom's voice was in my ear, and by Sunday evening, it had begun to sound like reason.

***

By the time Becky's car pulled into the driveway Monday afternoon, I had worked myself into something I am not proud of.

I saw her car, and I felt it, not warmth, not gratitude, but a hot, tight suspicion that had no real foundation and yet felt completely real. Tom's words had been turning in my head for two days, and by now they had become something that felt like my own thoughts.

Becky got out of the car and opened the back door for Chason. He looked better. His color had come back. He was carrying his bag, and Becky had her hand at his back, steering him gently.

"He did beautifully," she said, smiling. "Ate two bowls of soup last night. You would have been so proud. Here..." She reached into the bag and produced the bottle of amoxicillin. "One bottle down, he'll need to finish the course."

I looked at the single bottle.

And something in me that should have said *thank you* said something else entirely.

"Why is there only one bottle?"

Becky blinked. "The prescription was for one bottle, Tera. That's what they prescribed."

"You should have gotten more. What if he needs more?"

I heard my own voice, and some distant part of me recognized that it was wrong, that the sharpness in it was not about medicine at all. But I could not seem to stop it.

Becky looked at me quietly. "Do you want me to go back and..."

"You should have thought of it yourself!"

The words came out louder than I intended. Chason looked up at me, startled, still holding his bag.

Becky stood very still. The smile had left her face, replaced by something I had never seen there before in all my years of knowing her. Not anger. Something quieter and much harder to look at. Confusion. And beneath it, hurt as she had tears in her eyes.

"Tera," she said, carefully. "I paid for the visit. I paid for the prescription. I kept him all weekend so you could go to work. I don't..." Her voice caught for just a moment. "I don't understand what I've done wrong."

I reached past her and took Chason's hand, pulling him toward me.

"Just leave it," I said.

Becky looked at me for a long moment as a drop of tears rolled down her face.

Then she got back into her car.

I stood in the driveway and watched her drive away. Chason stood beside me, his bag in his hands, not saying anything.

The anger drained almost immediately. That is the thing about the kind of anger that does not truly belong to you; it does not stay. It burns fast, and then it is gone, and what it leaves behind is worse.

I thought about what she had done. The early morning call was answered without hesitation. The drive. The doctor's office. The shot and the prescription she had paid for herself. Two nights of soup and crackers and the particular comfort that only Becky knew how to give.

She had saved my job. She had cared for my son. And I had stood in my driveway and yelled at her about a bottle of medicine.

Chason was looking up at me.

"Mama?" he said softly. "Why were you mad at Grandma Becky?"

I could not answer him. I did not have an answer that was not an indictment of myself.

"Go inside and rest," I said quietly. "I'll bring your medicine."

He went inside. I stood in the driveway alone for a moment longer, the bottle of amoxicillin in my hand.

Tom had gotten into my head.

And I had let him.

That was the truth I could not escape, standing there in the afternoon sun with the car gone and the driveway empty. Becky had given me nothing but love, for as long as I could remember. Tom had given me suspicion and called it care. And I had chosen which one to believe.

I told myself I would call her. That I would explain. That she would understand.

But I did not call. Not that day. Not for a long time after.

And Becky, who had never once stopped loving me, waited.

A HOME

Tom continued to comment that he was saving toward getting me the home I wanted. His actions, however, spoke volumes. He was spending upward of $500.00 a month to rope in the local events. I would go with the boys and sit on the bleachers to watch him throw ropes at the calves' legs, working with a partner in the arena. He justified spending the money by saying he was hoping for the big prize of a horse trailer. I seemed to go along with his tales of less money now for more money later. He never won a horse trailer. He did win a buckle or two and once a saddle. None of that, however, helped toward a home.

Then, I became pregnant again. This was unexpected, not planned at all. At first, the news startled me, but once I adjusted to the idea of another child, excitement slowly filled my heart. The thought of a new baby brought a flicker of hope and tenderness back into my life.

I immediately called Becky and Penny, all excited about the coming birth. I asked Becky if she could assist with child care if I kept my job at the school. Becky was very happy to do so and even agreed to drive to my home to care for the baby.

That was the last Becky heard from me.

Becky tried several times to reach out to me, but to no avail. The silence that followed felt heavy and unsettling. She might have thought to herself that Tera will call when she needs me. I will wait.

Becky waited for Chason to call her, but he too went silent.

The silence from both of us left Becky with an ache she could not shake, as if something was deeply wrong and yet just beyond her reach.

On a hot summer night, I began to feel the first pains. I called my mother-in-law for a ride to the hospital. Tom was still working away from home and could not be reached. Finally, he called home after three days of silence. Where was he? What was occupying his time that made him unreachable when I was about to give birth? The questions settled heavily in my mind, but there was no time to dwell on them through the pain and uncertainty of the night.

Three days later, I called Becky to announce the birth of my little girl, Vickie. Vickie was a healthy baby, and everyone was excited to welcome her into this world. For a brief moment, the joy of new life seemed to soften the weight of everything else surrounding us.

School began in September, when Vickie was six weeks old and could be left, so I could go back to work. Work seemed to be my inner desire for freedom, even though it was still work. It gave me a reason to leave the house, a few hours where I could breathe beyond the walls of the trailer and the constant shadow of Tom's control.

I took Vickie to a local sitter. Becky was not called to babysit nor to assist in any way. Tom did not want Becky in our home. He claimed that it was too far for Becky to drive to be dependable. He had never been concerned before about Becky's travel time. The only reasoning I could come up with was that he feared Becky might influence me in some way to truly see my situation. Separation was still part of his game, and he was careful to keep those who loved me at a distance.

Chason was still attending the football games, still supporting the team, and still waiting patiently for his turn to play. Becky and the ladies at the orphanage came to every game, cheering and calling out his number with pride. He always knew they were there. After the game, he would meet them at the fence, speak for a brief moment, receive a hug, and then be gone again. To the ladies, those three short minutes were worth every moment of the long wait and every mile of the drive.

"I hope he knows how much he means to us," they would say. They had to drive an hour and a half back to the orphanage, traveling on very dark, unlit roads to get there, but no one minded that. Their love for him made every trip worthwhile, and each hug they received from him was treasured.

Christmas came around, and Vickie was now over three months old. The orphanage was lit up with lights, the walkway glowing warmly with Christmas lights along the trail. The great cedar outside was full of sparkling, twinkling lights that gave a sense of joy, peace, and excitement. It was a place filled with warmth and memories, and for me, it still felt like home in so many ways.

I arrived with the boys and Vickie. It was the first time that the ladies got to see and hold her. Everyone had a homemade gift just for Vickie, lovingly wrapped and prepared with excitement. The boys were not slighted. They too received gifts, ones that everyone hoped a teen would love to have.

Everyone passed Vickie around, cooing to her, singing softly to her, and praising her sweet little face. What everyone noticed, but kept their comments to themselves, was that this child did not look like me. She strongly resembled Tom's family genetically, with little resemblance to me at all. That realization brought a quiet disappointment to some because I was so beautiful. The baby did not carry those same features. Still, she had the sweet, innocent aura that only a baby can have, and that alone filled the room with tenderness and love.

I was asked again and again to make an effort to visit, to stay in touch. I seemed to be withdrawing more each time the ladies saw me. With every passing visit, I appeared a little farther away, a little quieter, and less like the bright young woman I had once been. They began to feel helpless, as though they were watching someone they loved slowly disappear behind a wall they could not reach through.

The following year, Chason saw Becky while shopping for school supplies. He told her that he had dropped football. It was the beginning of his third year, so it did not make sense that he would withdraw now, especially after waiting so long and being so patient for his chance to finally play.

"Why did you drop your favorite sport?" Becky inquired.

Chason answered with a defeated look, "I was told I was not competitive enough."

Becky responded, "Why would someone say that to you? A good teacher would never discourage a student that way. Who said that to you, and why are you listening?"

She knew that he did not have to answer. She could see it in his face, in the way his eyes lowered and his shoulders seemed heavier than a young boy's should ever be. Only someone with an evil motive would do that to a child who had finally found a sport, an outside interest, and something that gave him purpose. To take that away from him felt cruel, as though someone had intentionally dimmed one of the few lights in his life. It had to be someone who did not carry the love of a child in their heart.

They stood there in the school supply aisle for a moment longer. Becky did not want to let him walk away without leaving him with something to hold onto.

"Chason," she said. "Listen to me. Someone telling you that you are not enough does not make it true. Do you hear me?"

He looked at her. That same steady, too-old gaze.

"I hear you, Grandma."

"Good." She straightened up and held his face in both hands for just a moment, the way she had done with children at the orphanage since before he was born. "You are enough. You have always been enough. Don't you let anyone take that from you."

He nodded. She let go. He picked up a notebook from the shelf and placed it in his basket, and they said their goodbyes the way people do when they are both pretending the moment is ordinary.

It was the last time she saw him for a very long time.

There was no more contact with Chason after that. No way to see him now. The brief chance meeting in the store became the last thread, and once it was gone, Becky and the ladies at the orphanage were left with worry, unanswered questions, and the painful silence that followed.

A kind of emotional captivity was developing fast now within me and possibly within Chason as well. I was not acting like the Tera I once knew anymore. I was a different person, one shaped by fear, control, and years of emotional erosion. There was not a smile left that was not forced, and even those seemed faint and fleeting. Chason, too, was becoming a product of that same illness, learning to live inside silence and survival.

What would it take to change the situation?

CHAPTER FIVE

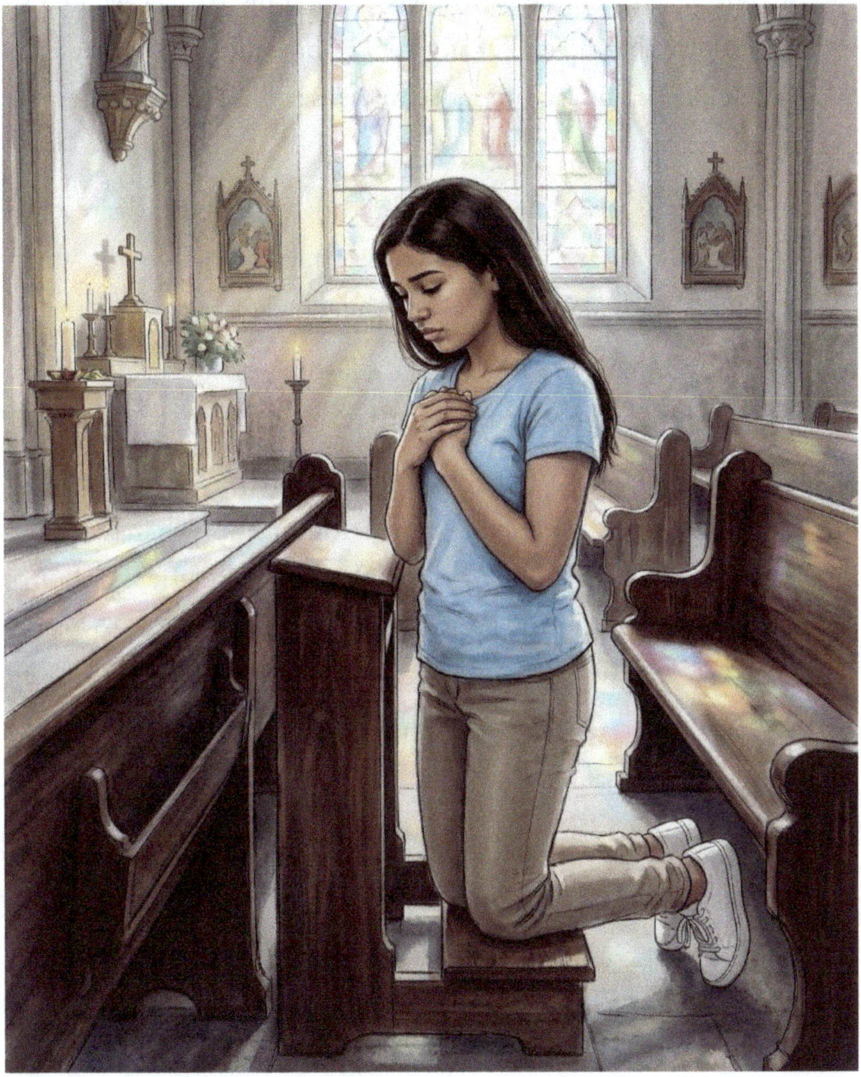

The church had become very important to me. I had convinced Tom to attend church with me. He went, maybe to win the battle, but the war was still ongoing.

He fulfilled his 'Christian' obligation, attending Sunday church whenever he was home. He even went down to the altar with me when I went. With each visit, he was slowly gaining my trust. I wanted so badly to believe that he had changed, that he could be sincere. Each Sunday felt like a small victory, a fleeting sense of hope that maybe our lives could improve.

One Sunday, as we walked back from the altar together, he reached down and took my hand. His grip was warm and steady in the way it had been in the early days, before everything had revealed itself.

"Do you feel that?" he asked quietly, leaning close so only I could hear. "That's real. What we have. That's real, Tera."

I looked straight ahead at the rows of pews and the soft light coming through the windows. Part of me wanted nothing more than to believe him. Part of me had heard those exact words before, in different rooms, at different turning points, every time I had come close to seeing clearly.

"I know," I said. Because it was the only answer I could give that would keep the peace.

And for a moment, walking down that aisle in the quiet of the church, I almost meant it.

Friends that I had formed over the years would suddenly stop visiting. Most of my social connections were tied to work or to church. No one wanted to come to my trailer. No one cared for Tom, and slowly the isolation started to press down on me, though I tried not to acknowledge it.

Time passed, but then an event occurred. Papa Tom came up with another idea, one that was still aimed at convincing me he was sincere in his promises to give me a home. We had been married now for eight years, yet I was still living in the small, single-wide trailer.

His idea? "I'll move the hay house over here and remodel it!" he said. What? He began to clear a spot for the house, just ten feet in front of the trailer. By adding onto the hay house, it would stretch to about seventy-five feet in length, completely blocking the trailer from view.

I stood at the kitchen window watching him pace out the ground with long strides, measuring with his steps as if the vision were already built.

"Ten years," he said that evening, setting his fork down and looking at me with the expression he reserved for moments he wanted to seem generous. "Ten years and it'll be everything you ever wanted."

I kept my eyes on my plate. Ten years. Chason would be grown and gone by then. I understood, in the quiet part of my mind that I did not often let speak, exactly what that meant.

"What does it look like?" I asked. "When it's finished. What does it look like?"

He smiled and began to describe it, room by room, with the easy confidence of a man who had done this before and knew I would listen. I sat across from him and nodded in the right places, watching his hands move as he spoke, and I thought:

I have heard this before. And I am listening again.

That thought came and went like a bird at a window. I did not hold onto it. I was not ready to.

He did just that. A moving truck pulled the hay house over and placed it carefully on the piers. The structure had been donated by his parents, and now it was under his control.

There would be a lot of work required to make that house a home. He set a goal of finishing it in ten years. Why ten years? Because by then, Chason would graduate. Tom had no intention of ever allowing his stepson to truly enjoy that home he claimed to be building for us. That was his plan, his hidden motive, carefully wrapped in the guise of generosity and care.

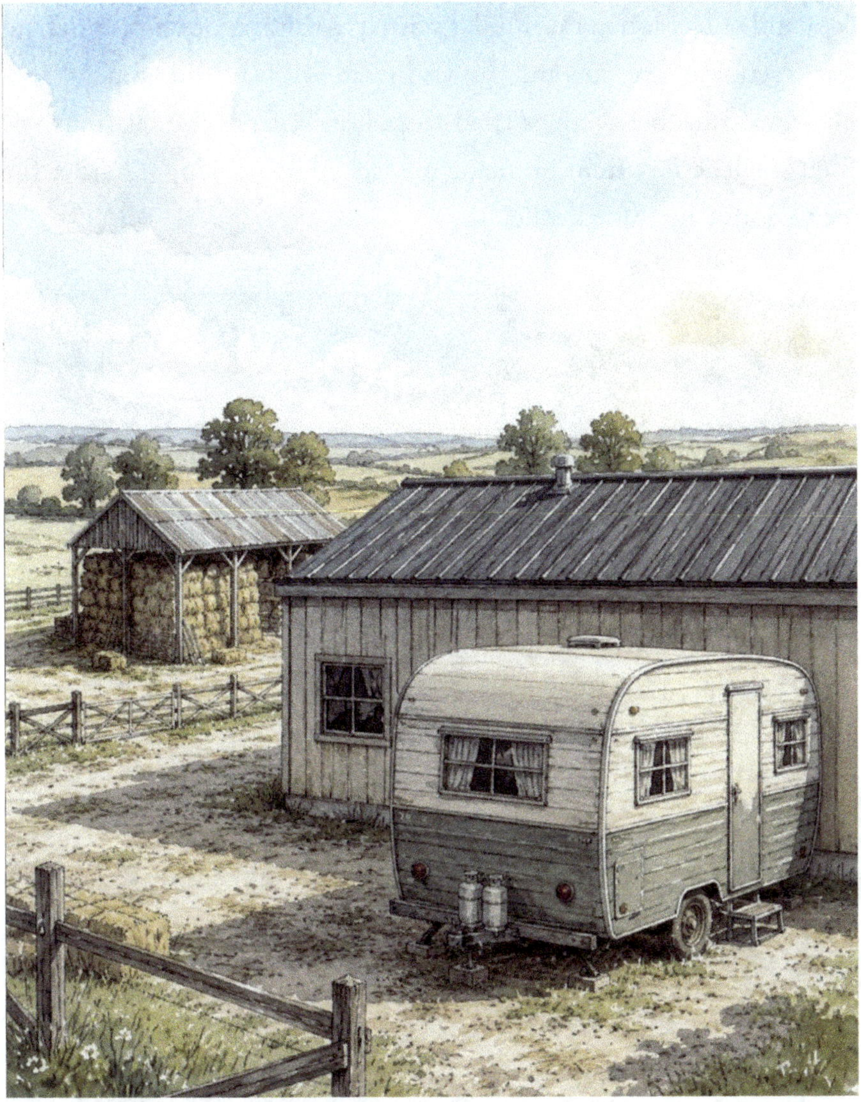

I was now living in a trailer facing the back side of this new building, completely blocking my view of anything but the hay house. Yet I smiled and went on, quietly accepting my situation. I seemed to have given up, resigned to whatever he did as being alright. The surprise bouquets, the occasional weekend getaways, they created a sense of debt and obligation in my mind. I started to think about how much he was spending on me and how ungrateful I would appear if I questioned his behavior or tried to pull back from the relationship. Each small act of attention made me feel guilty, making it harder for me to doubt anything he did.

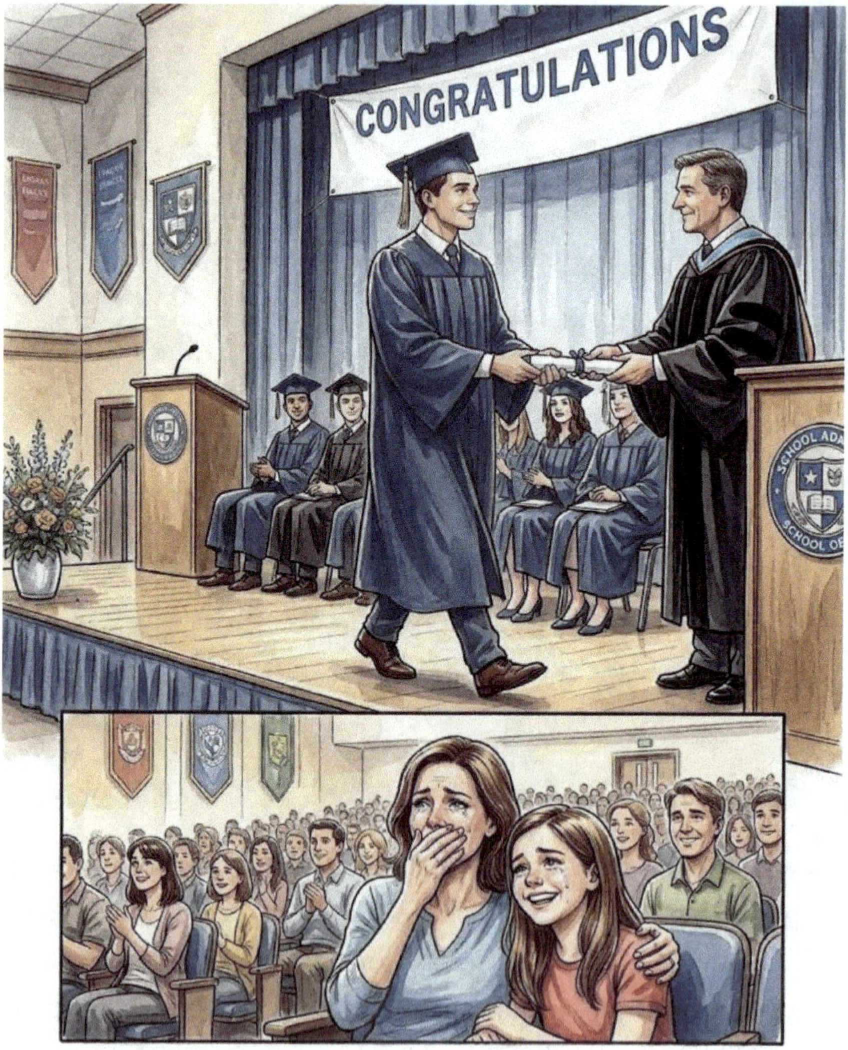

Chason soon graduated. Becky and Penny attended the ceremony, their hearts full of pride and concern for the young man they had watched grow through so many challenges. Chason walked down the aisle to receive his diploma, each step measured yet confident, carrying the quiet pride of someone who had endured more than most his age. As he moved across the stage, he spotted Becky in the crowd and lifted his hand slightly to wave. Becky smiled, a mixture of relief and happiness washing over her. Her favorite child was going to be alright, in spite of every obstacle he had faced.

After the ceremony, Chason met me, and together we went to a nearby restaurant to celebrate his accomplishment. I pretended not to see Becky and Penny. I was with Bubba and likely did not want to create any tension at home by inviting them along. Becky and Penny left the restaurant quietly, carrying a gift for Chason that they were unable to give him. Their hearts ached with hope and worry, believing that Chason would eventually reach out to them, reconnecting with the people who had always cared for him.

They did not speak until they reached the parking lot. The evening air was warm and still, and the sound of voices and music drifted faintly from inside.

Penny held the wrapped gift against her chest with both arms. "She saw us," she said quietly. It was not a question.

"Yes," Becky said.

"And she..." Penny stopped. She did not finish the sentence.

Becky opened the car door and stood there a moment before getting in, her eyes moving back toward the restaurant window where the warm glow of lights and the shapes of people could just be seen. Somewhere in there, Chason was sitting with his diploma and his mother and the man who had taken everything from both of them, piece by piece, year by year.

"We leave it," Becky said at last. Her voice was steady, though Penny could see what it cost her. "We leave the gift at the desk for him on the way out, and we leave the door open. That's all we can do."

"Do you really think he'll come back?" Penny asked.

Becky was quiet for a long moment. Then she said, "I raised that boy to know the difference between a cage and a home. Sooner or later, he'll remember."

They left the gift at the front desk with his name written on the card in Becky's careful handwriting. Then they drove home in the dark, not saying much, the road unrolling ahead of them like something that had to be gotten through before morning.

***

Chason turned eighteen while completing his studies. He now faced a future full of possibilities: college, a job, or whatever path he chose to follow. Finally, he had the opportunity to leave his past behind and start the life he had always dreamed of, free to make decisions for himself and pursue his own goals without interference.

Meanwhile, the hay house was not finished enough for us to move into. Tom claimed that money was short and we would 122 have to work on it as money became available. However, he did not let 'roping' interfere with lack of money. He paid as much as 500.00 entrance fee to rope once a month. That was money that could have been applied to having the home he had promised a long time ago. But nothing was said.

Chason now had the entire summer to think about his life and the choices ahead. He moved in with his father and Mimi, but when he did not call Becky after graduation, she began to worry that Stockholm Syndrome may have taken hold in him. She hoped that living full-time with his father would give him the clarity to recognize that something was not right and help him begin to think for himself again, reclaiming the independence and self-awareness he had been denied for so long.

Tyler, on the other hand, seemed fully immersed in life outdoors. He was taught to use a gun and often went hunting during deer season, sometimes bringing home a deer to be cured and prepared for eating. His life revolved around outdoor activities, hunting, fishing, and exploring the land around them. He sometimes played baseball, though he was not consistent enough to be counted on during games. Whether he attended or not, his focus remained on the things he loved, carving his own path in ways that were natural to him, free from the pressures and manipulations that had shaped his brother's early years.

***

LOVE BOMBING

Chason was out of the home. I found myself alone with my thoughts, reflecting back to the very beginning of it all. That first month had felt like magic, a moment I would never forget. Finally, someone had truly seen me, the way I had always longed to be seen. Years of feeling invisible, overlooked, and unimportant had left their mark on my heart. I had grown up in the orphanage, cared for but never fully belonging to anyone, watching other children get adopted while I remained behind. That constant waiting and longing had created a deep hunger inside me, one I had barely recognized even now.

The man who had swept me off my feet sixteen years ago knew exactly what he was doing. He had showered me with flowers, sent constant calls and texts filled with promises of love, and made me feel like the most special woman he had ever met. That rush of attention hit my heart like a flood on parched ground, filling spaces I had long forgotten existed. Every thoughtful gesture, every whispered compliment, was designed to make me feel extraordinary, chosen, and irreplaceable.

***

REFLECTION

Love bombing works because it targets the exact wounds that make a person most vulnerable. It is precise, intentional, and devastatingly effective.

When someone grows up without consistent parental love, their brain develops differently around attachment and recognition. Their nervous system becomes hyper-aware, constantly scanning for signs of acceptance or rejection. This sensitivity is both a superpower and a weakness. It allows them to care deeply for others, to feel empathy in ways most people cannot, but it also makes them light up like a Christmas tree when someone gives them the focused attention they have craved for a lifetime. The experience feels intoxicating, impossible to resist, and yet quietly dangerous.

To understand the process, consider this: the predator studies you carefully during those first few conversations, listening intently for clues about your past, your fears, your unfulfilled needs. He learns about the orphanage, about feeling different from other children, about the lingering questions surrounding your birth parents. He files away every detail of my longing to belong, to be chosen, to be loved unconditionally. Then, he becomes the person who seemingly chooses me above everyone else, at least in the beginning, creating the illusion of safety, trust, and unconditional devotion.

In those early days, every gesture felt miraculous to me. Every smile, every word of affection, every promise seemed to heal a part of my soul that had long been aching. And in truth, it did, temporarily. But it was the beginning of a pattern that would later manipulate my deepest vulnerabilities, weaving desire, hope, and love into a web I could not yet see.

If I could sit across from the girl I was then, I would take her hands in mine and say:

"I know how good it feels. I know that no one has ever looked at you quite like this before, as though you are the only person in the room, in the world. I know that it fills something in you that you did not even have a name for. You have waited your whole life for someone to choose you, and here he is, and it feels like the answer to every prayer you have ever whispered in the dark.

"But listen to me. Real love does not rush. It does not need to. Real love is patient because it is not afraid of what time might reveal. What you are feeling right now is not love growing. It is a door being forced open. And what comes through a door that is forced open is not what was meant to enter.

"You are not broken for believing him. You were made to love, and he found that and used it. That is not your failure. That is his.

"Trust the quiet voice. The one you keep pushing aside because it does not fit the story you want to be living. That voice is not fear. That voice is wisdom. And it has been trying to protect you from the very beginning."

I did not know any of that then. But I know it now.

***

Love bombing follows a specific pattern that feels natural, almost effortless, yet moves far too quickly to be genuine. Real love grows slowly over time, as two people gradually learn about each other, understand each other's fears and dreams, and build trust step by step.

Love bombing bypasses all of that. It skips past the normal stages of getting to know someone, rushing straight into declarations of devotion.

During this initial period, my brain released massive amounts of dopamine and oxytocin, creating a chemical addiction to his attention, validation, and approval. These are the same chemicals released during drug use, which explains why losing his focus or attention later felt like actual withdrawal.

The orphanage had given me love, but it was shared among many children and caregivers who eventually had to let me go when I aged out. He promised that I would never have to share his love or worry that he would leave. He made it feel as though I was the only person who mattered, the only one who could ever truly be understood and cherished.

The gifts, grand gestures, and constant attention served a specific purpose beyond simply impressing me. Every expensive dinner, surprise bouquet, and weekend getaway created an unconscious sense of debt and obligation in my mind. I began to think about how much he was spending on me, how much effort he was putting in, and how ungrateful I would be to question his behavior or pull back from the relationship. This is known as the reciprocity trap, and it works especially well on people who grew up feeling like they owed the world something simply for being cared for. Each gesture was designed to make me feel beholden, to blur the line between love and obligation, until questioning him or resisting felt impossible.

He isolated me from other perspectives right from the start, but it felt romantic rather than controlling. He wanted to spend every free moment together, making it seem as if his devotion was endless, when in reality, it was a calculated way to prevent me from talking to friends or family who might have noticed red flags. Whenever I mentioned other people in my life, he found subtle ways to point out their flaws or imply that they were jealous of my happiness. He especially targeted Becky.

The isolation crept in so gradually that I didn't realize I was losing my support system until it was already gone. By the time it became clear, the people who might have offered guidance, perspective, or even concern were distant, and I felt completely alone in my world with him.

The future planning began immediately, wrapped in a comforting sense of security after my childhood filled with uncertainty and instability. He spoke about marriage, children, growing old together, and all the adventures we would share as a couple. For someone who had never been truly chosen by a family, these promises felt like a miraculous gift, as if I had finally found a place in the world where I belonged. He painted detailed, vivid pictures of our life together, describing every milestone and every memory we would create, making me feel as though I was already fully committed to this future before I had the chance to really know who he was as a person.

My gut instincts tried to warn me several times during this period, but each whisper of unease was pushed aside because it didn't fit the fairy tale unfolding around me. Perhaps I noticed the way he spoke about his ex-girlfriends, or the subtle cruelty he showed toward waiters, or the sudden shifts in his mood when things didn't go his way. These little moments of discomfort were buried beneath the overwhelming flood of romantic gestures, declarations of love, and attention that made my heart race. I wanted so badly for this to be real that I ignored the warning signs, convincing myself that the magic was worth it.

But the warning signs had a way of accumulating, even when I refused to name them.

He had been with a woman before me. He had told me so himself, early on, in the careful way men introduce their past when they want you to know just enough to make them seem honest but not enough to make you ask questions. She had not been able to handle him, he said. She had not understood the way he worked, the long hours, the distance his job required. She had been insecure, jealous, difficult. He had used each of those words, and I had received them as warnings about her rather than reflections of him.

It was only later, much later, that I began to turn those words over like stones and look at what was underneath.

If she had been jealous, what had she been jealous of?

If she had been insecure, what had made her feel that way?

If she had not been able to handle him, what, exactly, had she been asked to handle?

Once those questions started, they did not stop. And quietly, without announcing themselves, they brought a new one with them.

If there was a woman before me, there might be one now.

***

He worked one hundred and fifty miles away. He had a mobile trailer at the job site. He was gone most of the week and only came home because he did not trust me, not because he missed me. Those two things had always sat uncomfortably side by side in my mind, but I had never followed the thought to where it led.

A man that suspicious of his wife is either that way by nature, or he is that way because he knows what people are capable of, because he himself is capable of it.

I began paying attention to small things I had previously let pass.

His phone is always face-down on the counter. The way he angled his screen when a message arrived. The calls he took outside, or in the truck with the door closed. The evenings when he was unreachable for an hour or two, and when I asked, the answer was always the same: work ran late, the signal was bad, he had fallen asleep early.

Each one, on its own, was nothing. Together, they were beginning to form a shape I recognized.

I mentioned it to Penny one afternoon, carefully, the way you test ice before you step onto it.

"Do you think it's possible," I said, "that he has someone at the job site?"

Penny was quiet for a moment. "What makes you ask that?"

"I don't know. Small things. Nothing I can point to directly."

"Tera." Her voice was measured. "You've been married to a man who checks your phone, controls who you call, drives three hours a day so he can watch you. What does that tell you about what he thinks people are capable of?"

I looked at my hands.

"That's what I thought," Penny said gently.

***

I chose a quiet evening to bring it up with Tom. Not directly, I had learned by then that direct questions were dangerous, that they gave him too much to work with. Instead, I moved toward it sideways, the way you approach a horse that is already nervous.

We were at the kitchen table after supper. He was reading something on his phone, which he turned over the moment I sat down.

"How are things at the site?" I asked.

"Fine."

"Getting along okay with everyone?"

He looked up. "What kind of question is that?"

"Just asking," I said. "You never really talk about the people you work with. I don't know anything about your days."

He relaxed slightly. This was a familiar territory for him, a wife wanting more communication. He could handle that. "There's not much to tell. It's work. You dig, you grade, you move to the next job."

"Is it mostly men on the crew?"

A half-second pause. Barely anything. But I felt it.

"Yeah, mostly. Why?"

"Just curious. Do you have office staff? Administrative people?"

Tom set his phone down and leaned back in his chair, and I watched his face shift into something more careful. The easy manner was still there, but behind it, something was assembling itself.

"Where is this coming from?" he asked. His voice was still even, still pleasant, but the question had edges.

"Nowhere," I said. "I just realized I've never seen where you spend your week. I don't know what the site looks like. We've been married, and I've never once visited."

He smiled then. It was the good smile, the one that had once made me feel chosen. "Baby, it's a work site. There's nothing to see. Dirt and equipment. You'd be bored in five minutes."

"Still," I said. "I'd like to see it someday."

"Someday," he agreed, easily, the way he agreed to all the things he never intended to do.

Then he picked up his phone again, and the conversation was over. He had moved through it the way he moved through everything, smoothly, without leaving anything I could take hold of. He had not answered the question I had actually been asking. But he had not panicked either, and I filed that away too.

***

I did not bring it up again.

I did not need to.

Because while he sat across from me thinking he had handled me, I was already making a different plan entirely.

He would not know I was coming. There would be no warning call, no careful preparation, no version of events arranged in advance. I would put the children in the car on an ordinary weekday morning, drive the hundred and fifty miles, and arrive at the work site the way truth always arrives, without an appointment.

I thought about the woman before me. The one who had been jealous and difficult and impossible to handle. I wondered if she had ever done what I was planning. I wondered if she had ever arrived somewhere and found what she was looking for.

I wondered if finding it had felt like relief or like the end of something.

I did not yet know which one I was hoping for.

But I was done waiting for answers he would never willingly give me. The girl in the red boots had climbed down toward the stage because she wanted something and simply went to get it.

It was time to remember how to do that again.

***

The love bombing phase typically lasts anywhere from a few weeks to several months, just long enough to get me emotionally invested and fully committed to the relationship. Once he felt certain that I was hooked, the behavior began to shift gradually. The constant texting became sporadic, the effusive compliments slowly turned into subtle criticisms, and the intense, focused attention was redirected toward other interests or distractions. By this point, I was already desperately trying to recapture those magical early days, trying to coax back the warmth and devotion I had fallen for, instead of recognizing that those days were never genuine in the first place.

AWAKENING

Understanding this pattern helps me see that the problem was never with me or my worthiness of love. I responded exactly the way anyone with my background would respond to someone offering what appeared to be unconditional acceptance and devotion. The manipulation worked precisely because it was designed to exploit my specific history and emotional needs. Recognizing love bombing for what it truly is gives me the power to protect myself, to regain clarity, and eventually to find the genuine, healthy love that I actually deserve. It is not a reflection of my value, but a reflection of how expertly the other person engineered the situation to draw me in.

I remember the exact moment when the fog began to lift.

I was sitting at the kitchen table on an ordinary Tuesday morning. Vickie was at school. The horses were quiet in the field. The house was still around me in the way that houses are when no one is performing anything for anyone.

There was a coffee cup in my hands and a patch of sunlight moving slowly across the floor, and I watched it the way I used to watch the horses from the orphanage window when I was very small, waiting for something I could not name.

I thought about Becky. I thought about Penny. I thought about the girl who had walked into a concert hall in red boots and climbed down toward the stage because she wanted something and simply went to get it, without asking anyone's permission.

She is still in here, I thought.

I did not leave that morning. Change does not often come in one morning. But something shifted, the way light shifts when a cloud moves, slowly at first, then all at once.

I set my coffee cup down. I looked at the sunlight on the floor.

And for the first time in a very long time, I thought not about what he had promised me, but about what I had promised myself, back before anyone had ever taught me to be afraid of my own wanting.

That is where the awakening begins. Not in the leaving. Not in the loud, dramatic moment of breaking free. It begins in a quiet room, on an ordinary morning, when a woman looks at the light on the floor and remembers who she was before someone else decided who she should be.

CHAPTER SIX

As soon as I began to feel and see this manipulation, I began to make plans. Plans that may not include Tom.

My son, Chason, had left our home. Asking him to come for a Sunday family dinner fell on deaf ears. He did not come to visit, always with an excuse to stay away. Sometimes he would suggest that we meet at a restaurant for lunch, rather than at the house. I noticed it but told myself it was just him growing up, finding his own way. Still, it stung every single time.

I remember one Sunday in particular. I had made a pot roast, the kind that took all morning, the smell filling every room of the hay house from six in the morning on. I had set the table for five, out of habit, the way I always did when I was hoping. I called Chason at ten o'clock, before church, to remind him.

"We're eating around two," I told him. "I made the pot roast. Your favorite."

"I know, Mom." There was a pause on his end, the kind that already had an answer in it. "I have something going on today. I'll call you later."

"Chason..."

"I'll call you, Mom. I promise."

He did not call.

I took his plate off the table and put it back in the cabinet without saying a word. Tyler watched me do it and then looked away. Even at his age, he understood that some silences were better left alone.

Tom was staying at work more, coming home less, which was suspicious. A far cry from the Tom of several years back. I began to wonder why. The romantic gestures were less. The phone calls during the day stopped. The little notes he used to leave on the kitchen counter were gone. I would sit at the kitchen table in the mornings, holding my coffee with both hands, staring at the empty spot where those notes used to be.

The change was not sudden. That was what made it so difficult to name. It had happened the way water erodes stone, so slowly, so quietly, that you did not notice until one day you looked down and saw that something solid had been worn away entirely. I kept asking myself when it had started, trying to trace it back to some turning point, some moment I could point to. I could not find one. It had not turned. It had simply faded.

One morning I sat at the table long after my coffee had gone cold, turning a small thought over in my mind that I had been trying not to look at directly for weeks.

He is different when he is here. But he is here less and less.

And when he does come home, he is already somewhere else.

I did not say this to anyone. Not to Penny. Not to Becky. I had grown so accustomed to carrying things quietly that I did not even notice anymore when I was doing it.

***

One weekend, I decided to travel to his work and spend time with him. Vickie was excited to get to go to her Daddy's workplace, excited to spend time fishing with him at the pond located on the job property. She packed her fishing rod, grabbed her hat, which was a special hat she wore that had fish hooks snapped into the band. It was a two-hour drive, so we left right after school let out, stopping just long enough to pick up travel snacks and food to attract the fish.

"Mama, do you think Daddy will be surprised?" Vickie asked from the back seat, her hat already sitting crooked on her head.

"I think he will be very surprised, baby," I told her.

She smiled and looked back out the window, watching the trees blur past.

"Will he be happy-surprised or mad-surprised?"

I glanced at her in the rearview mirror. She was looking at me with those wide, honest eyes that children have when they already half-know the answer to the question they are asking.

"Happy-surprised," I said, because she was seven years old and she deserved to believe that.

She nodded and pulled the brim of her hat down and went back to watching the trees. I kept my eyes on the road and tried to keep my own thoughts quiet.

We arrived at his mobile trailer close to 6 p.m. He usually finished his work at 4, so I thought this would be a pleasant surprise. His trailer had an outdoor cooking grill, so I had also brought steaks. I had packed everything carefully, thinking about how good it would feel to just sit outside together, eat a meal, watch Vickie fish at the pond as the sun went down.

It is 6 p.m. But no Tom.

I did not let him know we were coming, so I had not called him nor texted him. Maybe I should have, because he was not there.

Vickie jumped out of the car and ran to the door of the trailer, knocking hard.

"Daddy! Daddy, we're here!" She stepped back and looked at the windows. The lights were off.

I walked up slowly behind her and tried the door. Locked.

"Where is he, Mama?"

"I am not sure, sweetheart. Let me try calling him."

I began to call him, but there was no answer. I called again. Nothing.

Vickie pressed her nose against the trailer window, shielding her eyes with her hands to see inside.

"It's dark in there," she reported. "His stuff is there though. His hat is on the hook."

"Come away from the window, baby."

"Do you think he went to get something?"

"I think he must have," I said. "Let's walk down to the pond and wait for a little while."

Vickie's face cleared immediately, because the pond meant the fishing rod, and the fishing rod meant everything was still going to be fine. She ran back to the car for her tackle bag, already chattering about what she might catch, as if the evening had righted itself.

I watched her run and thought: she has been making the best of things her whole life. She learned that early, in this house. I did not know whether to be proud of her or heartbroken about it.

A LOVE BOMBER

When love bombing becomes the work of a predator, the pattern intensifies. My love bomber knew I carried a deep, unfulfilled well of longing inside me, an emotional emptiness that had never been properly nourished or validated. Tom positioned himself as the one person who finally understood me completely, who saw my true worth, and who promised to give me everything I had ever deserved. This felt like destiny because it spoke directly to the hunger that had been quietly gnawing at my heart since childhood. The intensity of his attention did not feel overwhelming; it felt like safety, comfort, and finally coming home after years of feeling invisible.

Tom counts on this internal dialogue, knowing exactly how to exploit it. He understood that women with abandonment wounds often preferred to ignore warning signs rather than risk losing what felt like their one chance at real love. He used my fear of being alone against me, making the relationship seem so perfect, so rare, that leaving became unthinkable. This is why love bombing is far more dangerous than simple manipulation. It weaponizes deep emotional needs, turning them into tools to control my own thoughts. It was a carefully orchestrated psychological campaign designed to make me emotionally dependent before I had a chance to recognize what was happening. The man who seemed too good to be true was exactly that, an illusion built to ensnare. The fairy tale beginning, with its flowers, declarations, and promises, was simply the setup for a nightmare I may still be living without fully realizing it.

It was not long before the cracks began to appear, small at first, almost imperceptible, but they grew steadily, eroding my sense of safety and trust.

I remember, once, describing to Penny the feeling I had during those early weeks with Tom. I had called her late on a Tuesday evening, Chason already asleep, the house quiet in the particular way it got at night.

"Penny, I feel like someone finally turned the lights on," I told her. "Like I have been walking around in the dark my whole life and I did not even know it, and now, now I can see."

"Just be careful you know what you are looking at," Penny said.

"What does that mean?"

"It means sometimes people turn the lights on so they can see you better. Not so that you can see them."

I had laughed and told her she was being dramatic. I was so certain she was wrong.

I have thought about those words many times since.

WHERE IS TOM?

When he didn't appear after a while, I thought maybe he had gone to the store. I walked back down to the pond where the kids were and found one of Tom's workers nearby. I asked him to keep an eye on Vickie for me.

"I just need to run and check on something," I told him. "I won't be long."

He nodded, and I got in the car and drove back to the trailer.

The man, his name was Randall, a quiet, sun-worn fellow who had worked for Tom several years, looked at me with an expression I did not quite know how to read at the time. It was not surprise at seeing me. It was something more careful than surprise. Later, I would think back on that look and understand it. He had known. Some of the men always know. And they are never the ones who tell.

"Is everything alright, ma'am?" he asked.

"Fine," I said. "I just want to check something at the trailer. I'll be right back."

He looked at Vickie, who was already crouched at the edge of the bank threading a worm onto her hook with the concentration of a surgeon. Then he looked back at me.

"Take your time," he said quietly.

The place was quiet when I pulled up. His truck was parked outside, which told me he was there. I sat in the car for just a moment, not really thinking about anything in particular, and then I got out and went inside.

The door was unlocked now. That registered but did not stop me. I walked through the small front room, the folding table, the two chairs, the radio he always left on, and moved toward the back, toward the rooms he used for storage and equipment. I was not looking for anything other than my husband. I just wanted to find him.

I pushed open one of the doors.

And there he was.

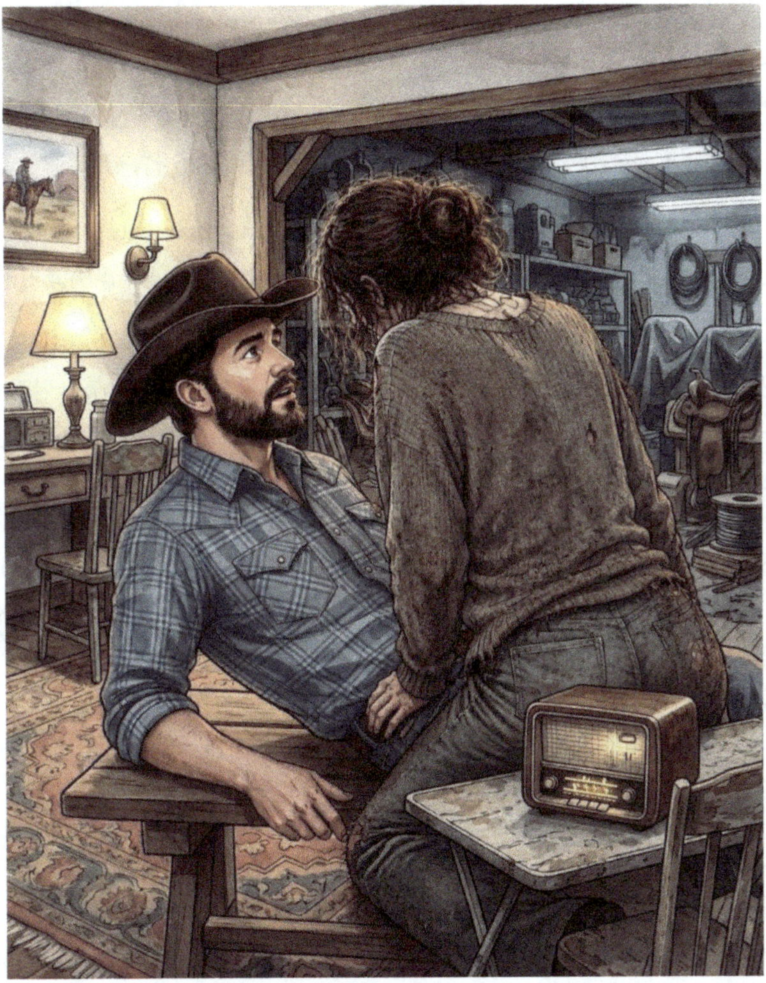

He was half lying across the table, and a woman was on top of him. I recognized her. I had seen her before, at a company event two Christmases ago. She had shaken my hand and smiled and asked me how I was enjoying the evening. For a split second, nobody moved. Then they scrambled. Tom pushed himself upright, and the woman stepped back, pulling at her clothes, and I just stood there in the doorway.

What surprised me most was what I did not feel. There was no gasp in my throat. No tears rushed to my eyes. No wave of shock rolled through me. It was as if some part of me had already known. As if my body had been quietly preparing for this moment for a long time and had decided not to waste any more energy being surprised.

I was sad. Yes. I will not pretend that I was not sad. But it was a soft, tired sadness. Not the kind that breaks you open. The kind that simply settles in and confirms what you already knew.

Tom cleared his throat. He straightened his shirt and looked at me with an expression caught somewhere between guilt and desperation.

"It is not what it looks like," he said.

Sixteen years of words. Sixteen years of the right phrase at the right moment. And this was what he had left. Five words that every person in that situation says, as though they are the first person to ever say them.

The woman said nothing. She had moved to the far side of the room and was staring at the floor. I did not look at her again. She was not the story. She had never been the story.

I did not say a word. I did not have any words for him in that moment. I turned and started walking out.

"Wait," he said. "Just wait, let me explain."

I kept walking. I heard his footsteps behind me, and then his hand wrapped around my wrist. He held it firm, the way he had held things in our marriage, like he had a right to them.

I jerked my hand away.

"Tera..."

"Do not." The two words came out very quiet and very final. I did not turn around.

"Please. Let me just, can you just stop for one second..."

"Let go of me, Tom."

He did. I do not know what he saw in my face in that moment. But he let go.

I did not yell. I did not turn around. I just pulled free and kept moving toward the door.

That moment, that simple act of pulling my wrist away from his hand, felt like more than just pulling away from his grip. It felt like pulling away from sixteen years of excuses, of looking the other way, of telling myself that things would get better. It felt like the door of a very long chapter clicking shut behind me.

I had no more reasons to stay. Not a single one. Whatever small thread of feeling or respect I had been holding onto for Tom was gone. I did not lose it in anger. I just looked for it inside myself and found that it was not there anymore.

I went back to get Vickie from the worker who had been watching her. She was sitting at the edge of the bank, her feet dangling, the fishing rod propped in her small hands. She had not caught anything, but she looked perfectly content.

"Mama! Come see! I almost had one. It tugged, and then it didn't tug, but Randall said that means they're interested."

I crouched down beside her and looked at the water. "That's good, baby."

"Did you find Daddy?"

I put my arm around her and pulled her close, and I pressed my cheek against the top of her hat. She smelled like sunscreen and pond water and something sweet she had eaten in the car.

"We need to head home, sweetheart."

She looked up at me. "What about the steaks?"

"We'll make them at home. It'll be just us girls tonight."

She studied my face for a moment with the quiet perception children have when they know something has changed but have not been given the shape of it yet. Then she turned back to the water.

"Okay," she said. "Let me reel in first."

She reeled in carefully, the way I had taught her, slow and steady so the line did not tangle. I watched her small hands work the reel and thought about all the things she did not know yet, all the things I was going to have to find the words for, all the explaining that was still ahead.

But not tonight. Tonight I would let her believe the evening had simply changed plans.

I loaded the car without much explanation, thanked Randall quietly, and I drove. I did not go back to Tom's place. I could not. The only place I could think to go was Chase's house.

Chase was not home when we arrived, which I was grateful for. I was not ready to explain myself to everyone all at once. But Chason was there, and when he opened the door and saw my face, he did not ask any questions right away. He just stepped aside and let us in.

"Hey, Vickie-bird," he said to his sister, using the nickname he had given her when she was a baby, the one that had stuck because she had been so tiny and bright-eyed. She brightened immediately and wrapped her arms around his waist, and he ruffled her hat and told her to go find the remote and pick something to watch.

Once she was settled in the other room, he turned to me.

"Mom." His voice was careful. Not alarmed, but watchful, the way it had been for years when it came to anything involving Tom. "What happened?"

I got Vickie settled, and then I turned to my son, and something in me gave way. I walked toward him, and I just started crying. Not the quiet kind of crying either. The kind that comes up from somewhere deep, the kind you have been holding back for so long that when it finally comes, it almost knocks you over.

He put his arms around me and held on.

"Mom," he said quietly. "Mom, what happened?"

I pulled back and looked at him. This boy of mine, who had been through so much. Who had grown up with Tom in the house, with all the tension and the coldness that came with that. Who had eventually stopped coming around altogether because being around us had become too painful. I had told myself for years that Chason was just being difficult, that he was just sensitive, that Tom was not as bad as Chason made him out to be. I had chosen wrong, over and over, and my son had paid the price of that.

"Chason," I said, wiping my face with the back of my hand. "I am so sorry. I am so sorry for everything you went through in that house. I am sorry I did not see it sooner. I am sorry I did not listen."

He shook his head slowly. "Mom, just tell me what happened. Did he hurt you?"

"Not the way you mean." I sat down on the edge of the couch and pressed my hands together in my lap. "I went to see him at the job site. Vickie wanted to fish at the pond. I brought steaks. I thought..." I stopped. Even saying it out loud, I could hear how it sounded, how I had talked myself into believing in a version of the evening that was never going to be real. "I thought it would be a nice surprise."

Chason sat across from me. He waited.

"He wasn't at the trailer when we got there, so I went to look for him. And I found him." I looked at my hands. "He was with a woman. In the back room."

The room went very quiet.

"Has Papa done something to you?" he asked, his voice low and careful.

"Not today," I said. "Not in the way that leaves a mark. But yes, Chason. Yes, he has."

I looked at my son for a long moment. He was not a little boy anymore. He had grown into a man who had learned early how to carry hard things. He deserved the truth. He had always deserved the truth.

So, I told him. I told him about driving to the job site, about Tom not being there, and about going to the trailer. I told him what I had found when I opened that door. I told him about the look on Tom's face, the words he said, and how I had pulled my wrist away and walked out without looking back.

I watched Chason's face as I spoke. His jaw tightened. His eyes went still and hard in the way that a person's eyes go when they are trying very hard to stay calm. By the time I finished talking, his hands were clasped together in his lap, and he was staring at the floor.

"I knew," he said quietly. "I knew something was wrong. I have known for a long time."

"I know you did," I said. "And I did not listen. I am sorry, son."

He was quiet for a moment. Then he said, "Do you remember when I was twelve and I told you he grabbed me?"

"Yes."

"And you laughed. You thought I was exaggerating."

The words hit me like cold water. Not because they were angry, his voice was not angry. It was simply matter-of-fact, the way a person speaks about a thing they have made their peace with. That made it worse somehow.

"I know," I said. "Chason, I know. I will carry that for the rest of my life."

"I don't want you to carry it," he said. He looked up. "I just, I needed you to know that I remember it. Not to hurt you. Just because I never got to say it out loud to you."

"You can say anything to me now," I told him. "Whatever you need to say. I am not going anywhere, and I am not going to look away."

He nodded slowly. The tightness in his jaw had eased a little.

"It is not your fault, Mom," he said at last. "You loved him. That is not something to be sorry for."

"I loved the person he pretended to be," I said. "I am not sure that is the same thing."

Chason thought about that for a moment. "Maybe not," he said. "But you didn't know the difference. That is not the same as being foolish. That is just being human."

We sat together for a long time after that, the house quiet around us, the little ones in the other room. There was grief in that room, yes. But there was also something else. Something that felt a little like relief. Like two people who had been carrying something heavy for a very long time and had finally, gently, set it down.

THE DAY I CHOSE MYSELF

Sitting with Chason that afternoon, something inside me began to rearrange itself. I started to see the full picture clearly for the first time, the whole lifespan of years laid out in front of me without the fog of hope distorting the view. I thought about my eldest son, who had grown into a man despite everything. I thought about my job, my income, my independence. I thought about who I had been before Tom, and who I had slowly been chipped away into becoming.

And I thought, maybe now. Maybe now is the time.

Chason was watching me the way he had always watched me, quietly and with great care, as if he were taking inventory of what I needed before I knew to ask for it. He had been doing that since he was small. I had not always recognized it for what it was.

"What are you thinking?" he asked.

"I'm thinking that I have been very foolish for a very long time," I said.

He shook his head. "You weren't foolish. You were hopeful. There's a difference."

"Is there?"

"Yes." He leaned forward, resting his elbows on his knees. "Foolish is when you don't care. Hopeful is when you care so much that you keep going even when you probably shouldn't. You cared, Mom. That's not a character flaw."

I looked at him for a long moment. I thought about all the times I had wished he would say something like that to me, and all the times I had not given him the opening to say it.

"When did you get so wise?" I asked.

He almost smiled. "I had a lot of time to think."

Because here is what I knew with absolute certainty in that moment: Tom was never going to change. Not for me. Not for our children. Not for anyone. I had given him every opportunity a person could give. I had prayed for it, waited for it, begged for it in the quiet of my own heart. And he had shown me, over and over again, exactly who he was. The problem was never that I had not seen it. The problem was that I had kept choosing not to believe it.

I was already too late. I know that. But I also know this: it is never too late to choose yourself. It is never too late to decide that you deserve something better than what you have been settling for. Every single day that I chose to walk out of that marriage rather than stay in it was going to be a day I gave back to myself.

I made up my mind to file for divorce. I also knew that it could be a problem.

But most of all, I knew that I could not leave my younger children, Tyler and Vickie, in that house. Tom had been decent enough to them, and I held no illusions that he was the same father to them that he had been a husband to me. But I had lived with Tom long enough to know that trust and Tom did not belong in the same sentence. I would be asking for full custody. I would be asking for child maintenance too, because those children deserved stability, and I was going to be the one to build it for them.

I said it out loud to Chason, not asking permission, but needing to hear myself say it.

"I'm going to file for divorce."

The words sat between us in the quiet room.

Chason looked at me steadily. "Okay," he said.

Just that. No fanfare. No long speech. Just the single word of a man who had been waiting for it for years, and who had the grace not to make that his mother's burden to carry.

"I'll need to go back to the house," I said. "To get our things. Mine and the children's."

"I'll come with you."

"Chason, you don't have to..."

"Mom." His voice was firm but not unkind. "I'll come with you. That's not a discussion."

I nodded. And I was so grateful I could not find a single word to say about it.

***

I went back to the house that same evening and started collecting my things. Chason came with me. He did not say much. He just showed up, the way good children do, and began helping me pack. Clothes, documents, the children's belongings. We moved through the house quietly and steadily, dismantling a life room by room.

I stood in the kitchen for a moment, looking at the narrow space I had cooked in for years, the plywood floor that had never been replaced, the window above the sink where I had once stood watching Tom pace out the ground for a house he had never intended to build. I ran my hand along the counter once, not with sentiment, only with the need to register what I was leaving.

Then I turned away and kept packing.

Tom was not there when we started, and part of me was grateful for that.

But then the door opened.

He came in fast, eyes wide, looking back and forth between me and the bags and Chason's expression. "What are you doing?" he demanded. "Are you mad?"

I almost laughed. After everything. After so many years of enduring, surviving, shrinking myself to fit into the space he allowed me. After that afternoon at the ranch. After every raised hand, every cruel word, every humiliation, large and small. He was asking me if I was mad.

I set down what I was holding. I looked at him, this man I had once believed was my great love, my fairy tale, my proof that someone could finally choose me. I looked at him, and I felt nothing that resembled love. Only clarity.

"I'm getting a divorce," I said. "It is over."

He stared at me. Something flickered across his face... surprise first, then the quick calculation I had seen so many times, the mental shuffling of which approach would work best here. The charming Tom or the frightening one.

"Now hold on," he said, and his voice dropped into the softer register. "Let's just talk about this. Whatever you think you saw today..."

"I know what I saw."

"Tera, listen to me. You are upset, and you have every right to be, but you are not thinking clearly right now. You are making a decision in the heat of the moment that is going to affect our whole family..."

"I am thinking more clearly than I have in all these years," I said. "And I have made my decision."

The softness left his face.

"You think you can just leave?" His voice had changed now, gone flat and cold in the way it did when he had stopped performing and had simply become himself. "After everything I have done for you? After everything I have given you?"

"What have you given me, Tom?"

He opened his mouth.

"A barn," I said. "A trailer. Blueprints for a house that was never going to be built. Phone calls sixty-three times a day. A night in a detention center. Years of promises that turned out to be nothing but air."

He stared at me.

"What you gave me," I said quietly, "was a very thorough education in what love is not."

And then I turned back to what I was doing.

That was the last time I ever needed Tom's reaction to tell me whether I was making the right decision. Because I already knew. For the first time in my life, I knew without needing anyone to confirm it for me.

His shock lasted only a few seconds before it turned into something uglier.

His face twisted, and he started yelling. Not the controlled, calculated kind of anger I had seen from him over the years, the kind he used like a tool to make me feel small and afraid. This was something rawer than that. This was the anger of a man who had just realized he was losing his grip on something he had always assumed was his to keep.

He stepped toward me, his hand coming up to push me back, his eyes hard.

And then Chason stepped between us.

I had not even seen him move. One moment, he was behind me, and the next, he was standing squarely between his papa and me, solid and unmoving, looking Tom directly in the eyes without a single trace of the fear that had lived in that house for so many years.

Tom froze.

The room went very quiet.

Chason did not raise his voice. That was the thing I would remember most. He did not shout or threaten or reach for anger the way Tom always had. He simply stood there and said, very calmly and very clearly:

"That's enough."

Two words. Quiet as a closed door.

Tom looked at him. I do not know what he saw in Chason's face in that moment. But whatever it was, it stopped him. He stood very still, and the muscles in his jaw worked, and then he looked away.

I stood behind my son and looked at the back of his shoulders, this boy I had held as a newborn, this child I had watched grow up inside a home that was never as safe as it should have been, and I felt something break open in my chest. Not grief this time. Something closer to wonder.

My baby had grown up. And he had grown up into someone who protected people. Someone who stood up when it mattered, even when it was hard, even when it was his stepfather standing on the other side.

Tom said nothing more. He knew, I think, that something had shifted permanently. He could not bully his way through this the way he had bullied his way through everything else.

We finished packing, and we left.

He watched us from the doorway as we loaded the car. I did not look back at him. I had looked back too many times already. I put the last box in the trunk, and I got in the driver's seat, and I pulled out of that driveway without a single glance in the rearview mirror.

Chason sat in the passenger seat and stared straight ahead. After a minute or two of driving in silence, he reached over and turned on the radio, low, and that was that.

***

After leaving the house that evening, I went straight to Chase's place. He had always been a decent man. Whatever had happened between us in the past, he had never been anything but good. Chase took one look at my face and asked no unnecessary questions. He let me in, made sure I was comfortable, and that was that.

I remember sitting on his porch that first evening, while the children were inside and the night had gone cool, and Chase came out and sat beside me without being asked. We had not spoken properly in a long time. Not since before Tom, really. There had been a distance between us for years that was made of too many things to name.

"You alright?" he asked.

"Getting there."

He nodded slowly. "Good."

We sat without talking for a while. The kind of quiet that is comfortable because it is between two people who have known each other long enough not to perform for one another.

"Chase," I said eventually.

"Yeah."

"I'm sorry. For a lot of things. For a long time ago and for after and for the parts in between."

He was quiet for a moment. "You don't need to apologize to me, Tera."

"I think I do."

"Then I accept it," he said simply. "And I'm sorry too. For the things I could have done differently."

I looked at him. "We were both very young."

"We were," he agreed. He leaned back in his chair. "We did the best we could with what we knew."

"I think that's the most generous thing anyone has ever said about my twenties."

He laughed, and I laughed too, quietly, and it surprised me... not the laughter itself, but how much it still felt like relief.

But of course, Tom, being Tom, did not simply let it go. He never could. Over the days that followed, he cycled through every strategy he had ever used on me. First came the anger, the phone calls full of threats and accusations. Then came the guilt, long messages about how I was destroying the family, how I was being selfish, how the children would suffer because of my choices. Then came the softer approach, promises that he had changed, that he understood now, that things would be different.

I listened to none of it.

Penny called me on the third day.

"He texted me," she said. "Asking me to talk to you."

"What did you say?"

"I told him I had nothing to say to him and he should direct all future communication to your lawyer."

I closed my eyes for a moment. "Penny."

"Don't you dare thank me. You know I have been waiting years to say that to that man."

I laughed, the kind of laugh that still has a little crying in it. "I know you have."

"Are you doing okay?"

"I am," I said. "I really am."

"Good." A pause. "Because I have blinds picked out for your new place. Whatever it looks like. I will bring them."

Not because I had become hard or cold. But because I finally knew the pattern by heart. I could see each move coming before he made it, the way you can predict the next line of a song you have heard a hundred times. This was not wisdom I had been born with. It was wisdom I had paid for, Sixteen years' worth of payments, and I was finally collecting what was owed to me.

I was not the old Tera anymore. The old Tera would have wavered. The old Tera would have heard his voice soften and felt that familiar pull in her chest, that desperate hope that maybe this time he meant it. But this Tera had seen behind the curtain. She knew what false love looked like. She knew what manipulation dressed up as remorse looked like. And she was done auditioning for a role in someone else's story.

This time, she was choosing herself.

***

I called Ms. Beth to began proceedings for a divorce. Chason came with me to every appointment, sat beside me through every meeting, and held my hand through the paperwork that slowly, officially, began dismantling a marriage that should never have consumed so many years of my life.

Then I remembered.. Something Tom said many years ago. He told me of his divorce from his first wife. He was bitter. He lost custody of his daughter. He never forgot what occurred before and during the divorce proceedings. He would make sure that never occurred again. Then he married me.

The opportunity came 6 months after our marriage when he tried to rape me, and then called the police to file the Domestic Violent charges against me. He knew that with a charge of violence it would be unlikely to issue custody to the parent with that charge, He knew exactly how to play the game, as he called it. I now would have to discredit him somehow. He filed a false charge , out of revenge, not of facts.

My attorney that represented me during the domestic charge will also represent me for the divorce. She met Tom then, and quickly assest him and his behavior and alerted me of his character then, I did not listen. I was in love, I thought. He told Ms.Beth that he would have the violent record explunged. But he never did and probably never intended to do so. It was his 'Ace in the hole'. He would have the upper hand in court.

Ms Beth called the DA , related the charges to him , explaining the circumstances. Now we would wait for the decision.

I had expected it to feel heavier. I had expected dread, or grief, or the particular shame of standing in an office and announcing to strangers that something you had tried very hard to make work had not worked. But it did not feel like any of those things. It felt like signing your name to something true. Like finally speaking out loud a fact that had been true for a very long time before anyone had said it.

"You okay?" Chason asked me quietly, on the way out of our first appointment.

"Yes," I said. "I am more than okay."

He looked at me sideways. "You sure?"

"Chason, I have been not okay for years. I know the difference."

He was quiet for a step or two. Then he said, "Fair enough."

We walked out into the daylight, and I tilted my face toward the sun for just a moment, and breathed.

I had expected him to be conflicted about it. But Chason was not. He was relieved. He had watched his mother endure for long enough, and now he just wanted her to be free.

I had filed for custody of Tyler and Vickie in the divorce, knowing that Tom may become a battle. But it wasn't. The DA granted a dismissal of charges immediately. The kids were still young, and they needed their mother. I told the court exactly that. I also asked for child maintenance, because my children deserved stability regardless of what their father had or had not done, and Tom was going to contribute to that stability whether he wanted to or not. The charges against me were dismissed as not valid. The DA took care of that after meeting Tom to discuss the situation.

***

For the first three days after leaving, I stayed at Chase's home. He even offered for me to stay as long as I needed, and I could tell he meant it genuinely.

But I said no.

I had just spent a life-time living inside someone else's space, someone else's rules, someone else's version of my life. I did not want to step out of one house and immediately into another. I needed something that was mine. Even if it was small. Even if it was bare. Even if I had to build it from scratch.

"You sure?" Chase asked, the morning I told him.

"I'm sure," I said. "But thank you. Truly."

He nodded. "You know where we are."

"I do," I said. "And that matters more than you know."

So I started looking for a place of my own.

I found it within the week. It was small, just two bedrooms, with no particular charm and no luxury to speak of. The kitchen was narrow. The living room could fit only the essentials. But when I walked through it for the first time, I stood in the middle of that small, plain space and I breathed. Slowly, fully, without checking over my shoulder.

It had peace. That was enough. That was more than I had had in sixteen years.

Penny arrived two days later with a carload of things she claimed she had been storing for me. Curtains, a rug, a set of kitchen towels in yellow, which she said was a color for new beginnings. She did not ask permission. She simply walked through the door with her arms full and started making the place feel like somewhere a person could live.

"I told you I'd bring blinds," she said, from the top of a step stool, already fitting them to the bedroom window.

"You did," I said.

"Are they the right size?"

"They're perfect."

She climbed down and looked at the window critically. Then she turned and looked at me.

"You look different," she said.

"Different how?"

She tilted her head, considering. "Like yourself," she said. "You look like yourself again."

I did not have words for what that meant to me. So instead I went and put the kettle on, and she folded the step stool back up, and we sat at the narrow kitchen counter and drank tea while the afternoon light came through the new blinds and laid itself across the floor in long, clean lines.

I could cover the rent with my salary. I had my job. I had myself. That was enough to build from.

Within a week, we were settled. Me, Tyler, Vickie, and Chason, all under one small roof, starting something new. The house was simple. Our evenings were quiet. There were no grand gestures and no performances. Just a mother and her children, learning what it felt like to exist without fear.

***

I remember sitting with the court papers in my hands and just being still for a long moment. Feeling no regret.

Tom had fought it the entire way. He pushed back on the custody. He brought up the false charges, but the DA quickly squashed the motion. He delayed things where he could. He made phone calls he should not have made and said things to people he should not have said. He was furious in the way that people are furious when they realize the thing they took for granted has finally stopped waiting for them. But I did not engage with any of it. I had my lawyer, I had

Chason, and I had a clarity I was not going to let anyone talk me out of.

My lawyer, a quiet woman who had heard every version of this story and still managed to treat mine as if it mattered, called me when it was done.

"It's official," she said. "How are you feeling?"

"Honestly?" I said. "Like I just put down something I have been carrying for so long I forgot what it felt like to have both hands free."

There was a brief pause on her end. Then she said, simply, "Good. That's exactly how you should feel."

***

A few months after the divorce, the child maintenance began coming through. Tom eventually approached the church requesting visitation rights with Tyler and Vickie, and the matter was brought to me.

I said yes.

I know that might surprise some people. But I was never trying to punish my children for their father's failures. Tom had not been a good husband to me, but Tyler and Vickie loved him, and they deserved the chance to form their own understanding of who he was. That was not my decision to make for them. When they were grown, they would make their own choices about how much of him they wanted in their lives. Until then, I would not be the wall standing between them and their father.

Tyler asked me about it one evening, the week before his first scheduled visit with Tom.

"Is it okay that I want to go, Mom?"

"Of course it is, baby."

"You're not mad?"

"Tyler." I sat down beside him and put my hand on his arm. "He is your father. I want you to know him. I want you to make up your own mind about who he is. That has nothing to do with me."

He looked at me, still uncertain.

"I am not going anywhere," I told him. "This house is yours. I am yours. You don't have to choose."

He exhaled slowly, the way children do when they have been holding something. "Okay," he said.

"Okay," I said back.

He went. He came home afterward and told me about it in the careful way he had, not wanting to upset me. I listened to every word and asked questions that showed I was interested, because I was. He was my son, and his life mattered to me, all of it, even the parts that included Tom.

Even Chason, as the years moved on, found his own rhythm with things. Some months he stayed with me. Some months he visited Chase. And I never said a word about it either way. He was a grown man making his own choices, and the greatest gift I could give him was the freedom to do exactly that, without guilt and without pressure from me.

I had spent so many years making myself small to fit into Tom's version of our life. I was not going to start controlling the people I loved just because I finally had the power to do so. That was never the kind of woman I wanted to be.

***

My world was small now, in the way that new beginnings always are. A small house. A modest salary. A handful of people I trusted. But for the first time, it was mine. Every corner of it, every quiet evening, every simple meal on that narrow kitchen counter. Mine.

I started reaching out to people I had let drift away. Becky was one of the first.

She answered on the second ring.

"Tera." Just my name, the way she had always said it, like it was something she was glad to have in her mouth.

"Becky," I said. "I'm sorry it took me so long."

"Oh, sweetheart." Her voice was warm and unhurried. "You're here now. That's what matters."

"I've missed you."

"I have missed you every single day," she said. "Now tell me everything. Start from the beginning and don't leave anything out."

I laughed. "Becky, it's a very long story."

"Good," she said. "I've been waiting a long time to hear it."

The speed of my fairy tale served a crucial purpose for the predator, which is why it prevented me from consulting friends and family who might have noticed concerning behaviors or questioned his motives. When someone sweeps you off your feet, declaring love and talking about marriage within the first few months, there is no time to introduce him to your support system or receive their honest opinions. By the time anyone who truly cared about me had a chance to intervene, I was already emotionally committed, invested, and unable to see the warning signs. After years, I stopped the Stockholm Syndrome (brain-washing) before it could take any more from me.

CLOSING NOTE

I want to say something to whoever is reading this, sitting with their own version of this story, their own Tom.

Healing is not a single dramatic moment. It does not arrive all at once, the way love bombing does, flooding you and overwhelming you and sweeping you off your feet. It is slower than that and quieter than that and, in many ways, far more real than anything I felt in those first dizzying months with Tom.

It looks like a small apartment with a narrow kitchen and not enough chairs. It looks like a phone call to an old friend you thought you had lost. It looks like your child standing between you and danger without hesitation. It looks like a piece of paper on a table that says, in plain legal language, that you are free.

It does not look like a fairy tale. But it is so much better than the fairy tale.

Because it is true.

I remember the morning after the divorce was finalized. I woke up early, before the children, before the light had fully come. I lay in my bed in that small, quiet house and I listened. Just listened. To the sound of nothing alarming. To the absence of dread. To the ordinary stillness of a morning that belonged to no one but me.

Then Vickie padded in from her room in her socks, her hair pressed flat on one side, and climbed up beside me and put her head on my shoulder without a word.

We lay there for a while in the early gray light.

"Mama?" she said, after a time.

"Hmm?"

"I like this house."

I put my arm around her. "Me too, baby," I said. "Me too."

I am Tera. I survived. I lost years I cannot get back, and I carry scars that did not exist before him. But I also carry something he could not take from me, no matter how hard he tried... the knowledge of my own worth, the certainty that I deserved better, and the proof, living and breathing and standing in my corner, that love, real love, had been around me all along.

I just had to get quiet enough to finally see it.

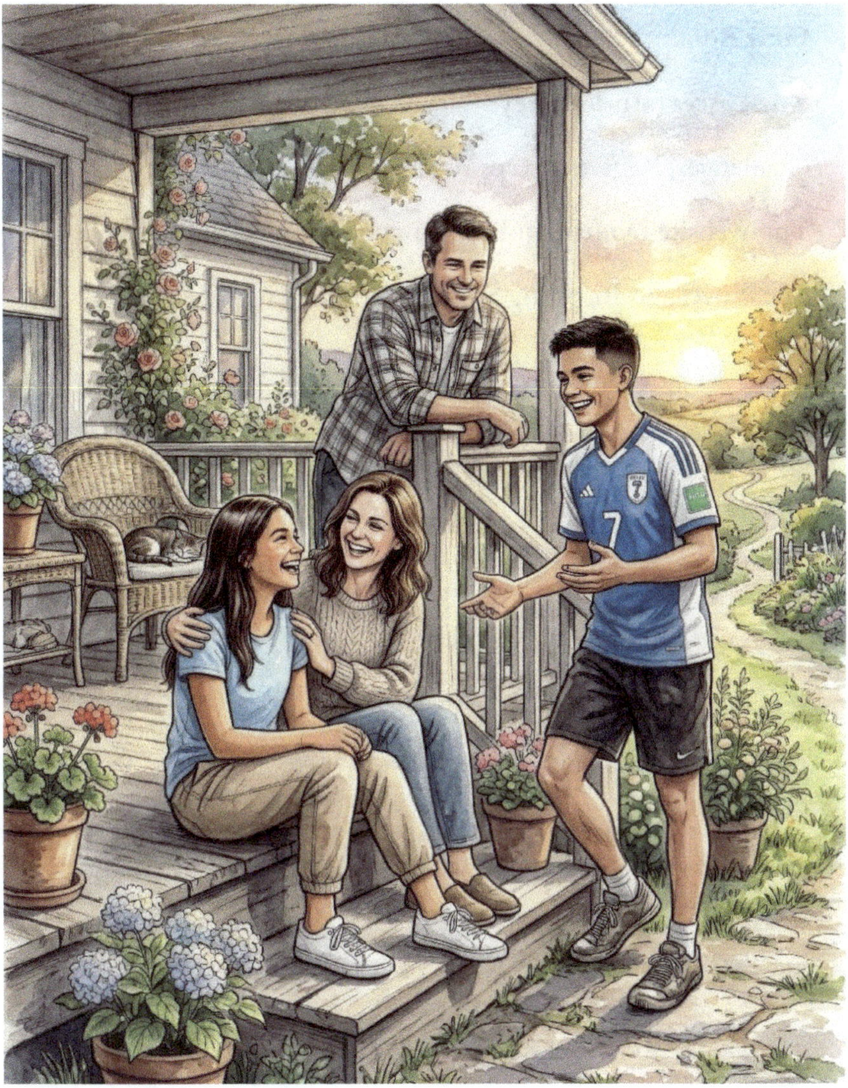

OTHER BOOKS BY THE AUTHOR

First Book:

The Uncertain Journey:

Challenges, Regrets & Opportunities.

The Website Domain: johnniehoggbeatty.com

Life, Love, and Inspiring Stories | Johnnie Hogg Beatty

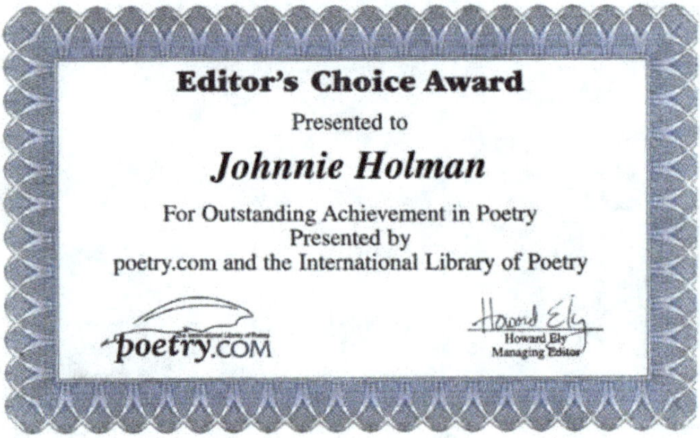

Second Book:

The Light

Web domain: johnniehoggbeatty.com

Inspirational-explores the journey of spirits to Earth, reflecting kindness and a sense of connection with the Divine.

www.ingramcontent.com/pod-product-compliance
Lightning Source LLC
LaVergne TN
LVHW022023051126
851858LV00003B/20
9781966606970